NURSING PROCEDURES

A Manual Used in the Teaching of the Principles and
Practice of Nursing in the Associated Hospitals
in the University of Minnesota
School of Nursing

By

MARION L. VANNIER

Director, School of Nursing, University of Minnesota

and

BARBARA A. THOMPSON

Supervisor of Clinical Instruction
Presbyterian Hospital School of Nursing, Chicago

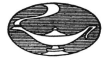

THE UNIVERSITY OF MINNESOTA PRESS

MINNEAPOLIS

PRINTED IN THE UNITED STATES OF AMERICA

TABLE OF CONTENTS
ELEMENTARY PRACTICAL NURSING

PREFACE

This manual of nursing procedures was prepared originally in mimeograph form for the use of students in the University of Minnesota School of Nursing. Soon requests for copies of the book came to us from various sources: from affiliating schools of nursing, from visitors and nurse educators, and from medical students and internes preparing for general practice.

The material, therefore, was carefully revised by a committee composed of instructors resident in the four associated hospitals of the University of Minnesota School of Nursing: Barbara A. Thompson, Instructor, School of Nursing, University of Minnesota; Lana Babcock, Instructor, Charles T. Miller Hospital, St. Paul; Minna Schultz, Instructor, Northern Pacific Beneficial Association Hospital, St. Paul; Melda Korfhage, Instructor, Minneapolis General Hospital, Minneapolis; Esther Andreason, Instructor, University Hospital, Minneapolis. After further testing, the manual was edited and rearranged for publication in its present form by Marion L. Vannier, Director of the University of Minnesota School of Nursing.

No attempt has been made to include any of the associated material given by the instructor in lectures preceding or accompanying the demonstrations. The purpose of the manual is to assure accuracy in detail and to obviate the necessity of note-taking by the students during the presentation of the demonstrations by the instructor. Harmer's *Principles and Practice of Nursing,* second edition, is the required text used in addition to this manual.

The arrangement of the material in lessons is in accordance with the plan followed in the University School. The students are taught first those procedures related to the patient's environment, then those minor duties affecting the patient which involve little responsibility, and gradually the student is taught, and allowed to carry out, the more difficult procedures.

The course covers eighty hours divided into fifty-two hours of Elementary Practical Nursing and twenty-eight hours of Advanced Practical Nursing. Thirteen two-hour periods are used by the instructor in presenting the lectures and demonstrations of the first part, and thirteen two-hour periods are used by the students in class practice, presenting return demonstrations for the instructor's criticism. The same arrangement is carried out with the fourteen lessons in the Advanced Procedures.

The four associated hospitals of the University School of Nursing are of widely different types and have a joint capacity of 1,292 beds. Because of the varied and complete services they offer, we believe that this manual of the procedures now being used in them will be found adapted to the use of other schools of nursing, connected with hospitals of various kinds.

The hospitals associated in the school are:

1. The Minneapolis General Hospital, with 525 beds, for the care of the indigent sick of the *city*.

2. The Elliot Memorial, Christian and Todd Memorial, and Eustis Building—units of the University Hospital, with 400 beds, for the care of the indigent sick of the *state*, the treatment of patients suffering with cancer, Students' Health Service, and out-patient clinics.

3. The Charles T. Miller Hospital, St. Paul, with 200 beds, for the care of private patients.

4. The Northern Pacific Beneficial Association Hospital, St. Paul, with 167 beds, for the care of private patients.

The Glen Lake Sanitorium, with 750 beds, for the care of the tuberculosis patients of the *county*, is affiliated with the School of Nursing.

MARION L. VANNIER
Director, School of Nursing,
University of Minnesota

ELEMENTARY PRACTICAL NURSING

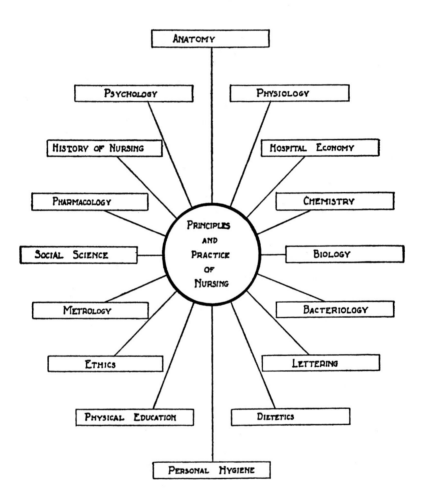

NURSING PROCEDURES

"Nursing procedures include all the simple duties of daily nursing care as well as the nursing treatments for the cure or prevention of disease which the doctor prescribes and for the performance of which the nurse is, usually in the doctor's absence, responsible.

"The teaching of practical procedures is thus in a sense the center of the nurse's training, the basis of her future professional usefulness. Indeed the 'theory and practice of nursing,' as this subject is usually called, is more far-reaching and inclusive than appears at first sight, for in it are practically all the other important subjects of the nurse's curriculum."[1]

Nursing procedures are to be carried out with the following points in mind:

1. The comfort and happiness of the patient, mental and physical.
2. The therapeutic effect of the treatment or service.
3. The safety of the patient, the nurse, and others.
4. The economy of energy, time, and materials.
5. Accuracy in detail.
6. Artistic, finished appearance of work.
7. Technique and dexterity.
8. Simplicity.

Reference books to be used in teaching the course:

Harmer, *The Principles and Practice of Nursing* (2nd edition).
Sanders, *Modern Methods in Nursing.*
Goodnow, *The Technic of Nursing.*
Kelley, *The Textbook of Nursing Technique.*

---

[1]*Rockefeller Foundation Report on Nursing and Nursing Education in the United States.*

LESSON I
CLEANLINESS AND ORDER
Care and Hygiene of the Ward

Aim

1. Cleanliness as a precaution against contamination.
2. Order as an aid to more efficient work.

General instructions

1. Always have a definite plan of procedure before beginning work in the ward.
2. Keep rooms or wards well lighted, but do not leave artificial lights on unnecessarily.
3. Care properly for the furniture, utensils, and linen.
4. Prevent noise.
5. While in room or ward always attend to the immediate needs of the patient.
6. Keep tops of stands clear for tray, drinking glass, and flowers.

Room or ward order

1. Keep room or ward clean and in perfect order.
2. Adjust window shades to uniform height; remove articles from sill at the same time.
3. Beginning at right side of ward:
   a. Remove utensils.
   b. Remove all refuse and place in paper bag or newspaper.
   c. Strip and make empty beds. Leave bed and chair straight, wheels of bed turned in, stand in order, and towels folded neatly before going to the next bed.
4. Do not permit an accumulation of articles on stands.
5. Do not leave articles on the radiators.
6. Do not put things between mattress and springs on the bed.
7. Always note when leaving room or ward whether there are any articles to be removed.

Room or ward hygiene

1. Keep room or ward well ventilated without allowing patient to be in a draft.
2. Prevent unpleasant odors by:
   a. Keeping the bed utensils clean and covering them as soon as you take them from the patient.
   b. Keeping all patients and their bedding clean.
   c. Flushing the toilets and the hoppers when necessary and keeping them in perfect order.
   d. Placing soiled dressings in the case provided for them as soon as you take them from the patient.

e. Changing the water on flowers daily.
3. Bed pans and urinals must not be placed on tables, chairs, or floor. They must be left in bed until taken directly to the lavatory.
4. Temperatures advised:
   a. General ward, 68° F.
   b. Bathroom, 72° F.
   c. Surgical department, 75° to 80° F.

Dusting and Cleaning

Aim
1. Cleanliness.

General instructions
1. Have the right attitude toward the work.
2. Dust after sweeping, not before.
3. Use clean water and a clean duster.
4. Use a damp (not wet) cloth, to which the dust particles will adhere, for all surfaces except electric fixtures and polished furniture.
5. Dust with a firm, even stroke, not round and round.
6. Dust thoroughly, especially in the corners.
7. Develop a system of working by which you avoid waste of time and energy.
8. Be economical in the care and use of materials.
9. Dust thoroughly every day.

Necessary articles
Basin of hot water.
Two dusters.
Soap.
Bon Ami cake or powder.
Newspaper.

Procedure
1. Fill the basin half full of hot water and carry it with the other articles to the room or ward.
2. Spread the newspaper on the bedside table and place the articles so that they will be convenient for use.
3. Dust the bed, table, chairs, and window sills. Pay particular attention to rounds on bed and chairs.
4. Dust, remove refuse, and straighten articles on bedside table.
5. Place all furniture in position, adjust the window shades, and carry cleaning articles to the service room.
6. Wash dusters with soap and water and hang to dry in the place provided for them. Leave other articles clean and in proper place.

Care of Service Room

General instructions

1. Pick up and put in proper places all articles out of place.

Procedure

1. Wash basins, mouth-wash cups, and emesis basins:
   a. Wash with cold water and boil after use. (Place all utensils upside down in sterilizer.) Always add 1 cup of Wyandotte's Cleaner to a sterilizer (large) of water, and ½ cup to small sterilizer when sterilizing utensils.
   b. Remove from sterilizer, wash with soap, water, Bon Ami, and dry.
2. Bed pans and urinals:
   a. Boil daily and wash with soap and water. Dry and place on rack.
3. Enema cans, pitchers, foot tubs, trays, vases, etc.:
   a. Wash thoroughly after use.
   b. Dry and replace on shelf.
   c. Boil when contaminated.
4. Hoppers:
   a. Flush.
   b. Clean with stiff, long-handled brush.
   c. Complete cleaning with cloth, soap, and water.
   d. Remove stains with Bon Ami or kerosene.
5. Faucets:
   a. Nickel—clean with soap and water or Bon Ami. Rub dry.
   b. Brass—clean with metal polish.
   Note: In using Bon Ami, be sure that all is removed with a dry cloth.
6. Table and utensil rack:
   a. Remove refuse and unnecessary articles. Wash and put clean paper on shelves and tables daily. Wipe off all bottles. Report empty bottles to head nurse.
7. Cupboards, drawers, shelves:
   a. Keep free of refuse.
   b. Clean daily.
8. Sterilizer, basin and instrument:
   a. Clean inside of sterilizer every Saturday. Use one cup of sal soda to ¾ sterilizer of water. If any sediment remains on sterilizer, apply dilute hydrochloric acid with a tongue depressor, swab and neutralize with ammonia. Remove all loose sediment. (It clogs the waste pipes.)

Care of Bathroom and Lavatory

Necessary articles

Two cleaning cloths.	Bon Ami cake or powder.
Soap.	Kerosene.

Procedure

1. Remove soiled towels, unnecessary articles, and refuse.
2. Clean the porcelain tub and wash bowl with either Bon Ami or kerosene, followed by hot water and soap.
3. Flush toilet and clean with hopper brush. Clean bowl inside and outside.
4. Dust furniture, and clean all utensils, etc., which are left in the bathroom.

Care of plumbing

1. Do not throw coffee grounds, hair, thread, cakes of soap, wash cloths, towels, matches, or anything that will not dissolve into hoppers, sinks, tubs, etc.
2. Report defects at once.
3. Never allow water to run or drip from faucets, as it results in an unnecessary waste of the water supply and unnecessary wear of the faucets.
4. Sal soda solution (dr. 12 to 1 qt. of water) can be used in waste pipes every few days to keep them free from accumulation of grease.

LESSON II

CLEANLINESS AND ORDER, Continued

Cleaning a Bed After Discharge of Patient

Aim
1. Cleanliness.
2. To have the bed ready for new patient.

Articles necessary

Basin of hot water.
Bon Ami cake or powder.
Soap.
Newspaper.
Whisk broom.
Two dusters.

Procedure
1. Carry articles to the bedside.
2. Remove the linen and place it directly in the hamper.
3. Hang the blankets over the back of a chair to air, or place them in the hamper with the soiled linen if necessary. (Consult head nurse as to the routine care of blankets.)
4. Dust mattress with dampened whisk broom. Be sure and get into all the crevices. Brush dust into newspaper folded as a cornucopia.
5. Turn mattress back on itself.
6. Dust one-half of springs and ledge underneath, head and foot.
7. Wash bed thoroughly.
8. Turn mattress back on clean half of springs.
9. Place rubber sheet across springs.
10. Wash rubber sheet. Use Bon Ami to remove stains.
11. Turn rubber sheet back upon mattress, soiled side of rubber sheet out.
12. Wash other half of springs.
13. Place rubber sheet on springs, soiled side out.
14. Wash rest of rubber sheet.
15. Wash bedside stand and chair.
16. Air bed as long as possible (1 to 2 days).
17. Make up as a closed bed.
18. Leave bed, bedside stand, and chair complete and ready for a new patient.

Removal of Stains[1]

Blood
1. Fresh blood:
   a. Soak in cold water.

---

[1] Reproduced by permission from the *Modern Hospital*, January, 1925.

b. Wash in soap and water.
c. Apply hydrogen peroxide.
2. Old blood:
   a. Keep wet with hydrogen peroxide and ammonia for several hours.
3. Thick blood on bed ticking:
   a. Apply a thick paste of starch and water and allow to stand for several hours in the sun. Apply fresh paste when this becomes discolored. (On blankets use same treatment, but wash with Ivory soap and water.)

Ink

1. When fresh, wash out in clear water.
2. Apply dilute oxalic acid, one quarter teaspoonful to one cup of water. Wash out with water and repeat if necessary.
3. Alternate potassium permanganate (1 gram to 1 liter of water) and oxalic acid.
4. Soak or boil in sour milk.
5. Soak in sweet milk.
6. Apply lemon juice and salt and keep in the sun.
7. Try ammonia and alcohol.
8. Ink on carpet:
   a. Apply dry salt and renew when stained.
9. Ink on wood:
   a. Apply oxalic acid.
10. Indelible ink:
    a. If base is aniline dye, it cannot be removed.
    b. If base is silver nitrate, apply a 10 per cent solution of potassium cyanide.
11. Ink eradicator.
12. Dakin's solution, soap, and rubbing.

Rust

1. Use salt and lemon juice, place article in the sun.
2. Apply oxalic acid or dilute hydrochloric acid. Wash out in water.
3. Try salts of lemon.

Fruit

1. Fresh fruit stains (except peaches):
   a. Rub stain with salt and apply boiling water.
2. Old fruit stains:
   a. Soak in weak oxalic solution.
   b. Bleach with peroxide and ammonia.
3. Peach stains:
   a. Apply alcohol.
4. Grape juice stains:
   a. Bleachers: oxalic acid, ammonia, or hydrogen peroxide.

Chocolate and cocoa stains

1. Cover with borax and soak with cold water. Pour boiling water through stain.

Coffee and tea stains

1. Ordinary laundering will usually remove stain.
2. Pour on boiling water from a height.
3. Apply dilute ammonia; wash when color disappears.
4. Use peroxide and ammonia for old coffee and tea stains.

Grease

1. Cannot be removed if washed in water.
2. Soak in kerosene before washing.
3. Wash with turpentine; oil may be absorbed by using blotting paper or powdered chalk.
4. Gasoline may be used for materials that cannot be washed.
5. Chloroform may be used. Always use in daylight and in a draft, and have several folds of cloth under stain.
6. Axle grease on linen:
   a. Grease well with lard or butter and wash in tepid, soapy water.
7. Tar:
   a. Use gasoline.
8. Glue:
   a. Soak in vinegar and wash in soapy water.
9. Grass stains:
   a. Soak in alcohol and wash in usual way.
   b. Apply lemon juice and salt and place in the sun.
10. Gum:
   a. Remove with ether.
   b. Alcohol.

Mucus

1. Wash in ammonia and water or in salt and water before using soap.

Perspiration

1. Use a strong soap solution and let the article lie in the sun.

Urine

1. Wash with warm, soapy water.
2. Sponge with alcohol.

Feces

1. Wash with cold water at once.
2. Allow to soak in cold, soapy water, and boil.

Mildew

1. Moisten with strong soap solution.

2. Apply a paste of soap, salt, and chalk, and leave in the strong sunlight for several hours; if unsuccessful, use Javelle water or other bleaching agent.
3. Try lemon juice and salt.

Milk or cream

1. Wash out with cold water and then with warm, soapy water.

Removal of Stains from Drugs

Coal-tar products

1. Try tincture of green soap.
2. Try potassium permanganate and oxalic acid.

Argyrol

1. Soak in 10 per cent potassium cyanide.
2. Use Dakin's solution.
3. Bichloride of mercury 1-500; rinse well.

Silver nitrate

1. Bichloride of mercury; rinse well.
2. 5 per cent potassium cyanide.
3. Remove from hands with potassium iodide solution.
4. Remove from linen with argyrol or bichloride of mercury solution 1-500; rinse thoroughly.

Acid stains

1. Neutralize with ammonia.
2. If acid has removed the color, it may be brought back with chloroform.
3. For a skin burn with acid, rinse with water immediately to dilute the acid, and apply ammonia.
4. In case of a phenol (carbolic acid) burn, apply alcohol at once.

Iodine

1. On linen:
   a. Fresh stains may be removed by washing in warm, soapy water.
   b. May be removed by boiling.
2. On wood:
   a. Cover with cold starch paste until iodine is absorbed and wash with ammonia and water.
3. On skin:
   a. Wash with alcohol.

Potassium iodide

1. Dakin's solution.
2. Alcohol.
3. Hot ammonia.

Potassium permanganate

1. Oxalic acid solution.
2. Hydrogen peroxide.

Oil

1. On linen:
   a. Use kerosene, then soap and water.
   b. Camphorated oil is removed with ether.
   c. Try turpentine on carron oil.
2. On marble:
   a. Wash with soda bicarbonate solution.
   b. Apply paste of ammonia and whiting and let stand for 24 hours.

Paint

1. Try benzine or turpentine.   (If dry, apply vaseline first.)

Bichloride of mercury

1. Soak in Labarraque's solution for several hours, then wash and rinse.

Balsam

1. Alcohol.
2. Bleachers.

Picric acid

1. Dakin's solution.

Mercurochrome

1. Dakin's solution.
2. Soap and water and rub.

Cod-liver oil

1. Carbon tetrachloride and follow with soap and water.
2. Acetone.

Extract of Hamamilis

1. Use a good bleach, for example, Javelle water.
2. Soap and water.

Tincture of benzoin

1. Javelle water.
2. Ammonia.
3. Hydrogen peroxide.
4. Alcohol.
5. Ether.

LESSON III

CLEANLINESS AND ORDER, Continued

Care of Rubber Goods and Glass Utensils

Aim

1. To prolong life of articles.
2. To put articles away in such a condition that they will be ready for use when needed.

Articles in common use in hospital

1. Gastric lavage tube.
2. Rectal tube.
3. Ewald evacuating bulb.
4. Rubber gloves.
5. Hard rubber goods (enema and douche tips, bougies, syringe, pessaries, catheters).
6. Rubber and silk catheters.
7. Silk ureter catheters.
8. Glass utensils (douche points, connecting points, etc.).

General instructions

Rubber appliances are expensive and need constant attention.

1. Never stick pins into a rubber appliance.
2. Oil and grease cause rubber to become soft and partially dissolved.
3. Acids corrode it.
4. Prolonged heat destroys it.
5. Folding cracks it. All rubber sheeting should be rolled or hung on bars.
6. If not used it becomes dry and should be soaked in cold water occasionally.
7. See that the rubber washer is on the stopper and cap of hot water bottle (caps, stoppers, and rings can be ordered when lost).
8. Hot water bottle stoppers can be attached to container with tape or string if necessary.
9. Clamps on rubber tubing should always be unfastened when not in use.
10. Tubing should never be removed from can. Drain well, coil loosely, never at sharp angles.
11. Hard rubber tubes should be allowed to cool immediately; care should be taken that they are placed in such a way as not to alter their shape while soft.

To clean

1. Clean immediately after using, with cold water.
2. Wash with soap and tepid water and rinse.
3. Wrap in muslin and boil for 3 minutes.

To mark

1. Use fresh stick of lunar caustic, slightly moistened.

When put away

1. All rubber should be dry.
2. Tubing should be straight.
3. Bags, air cushions, ice caps, etc., should be slightly inflated.
4. Gloves should be powdered.

Ewald evacuating tube and gastric lavage tube

1. Clean with cold water immediately after use.
2. Following are two methods for disinfecting. Use the one approved by the hospital in which you are working.
   a. Drop into boiling water for 2 minutes. Do not leave until you have removed the tube and bulb. Remove, dry thoroughly, and put away, being sure that the tubing is not bent.
   b. Place tube and bulb in a 2 per cent liquor cresolis compositus for 20 minutes. Remove and wash with soap and tepid water, rinse thoroughly. Dry thoroughly and put away; be sure that the tube is not bent.

Care of rubber gloves

1. Wash the gloves in cold water.
2. Wrap in muslin and boil for 3 minutes or drop into a disinfectant solution. (Use method approved by the hospital in which you are working.)
3. Wash both sides of gloves with warm water and soap.
4. Rinse and dry thoroughly.
5. Inflate them to discover holes and put aside all imperfect gloves.

Care of hard rubber goods

1. Clean immediately after use, with cold water.
2. Drop into boiling water for 2 minutes or disinfect with liquor cresolis compositus.
3. Wash with soap and tepid water, rinse thoroughly.
4. Dry and put away in container provided for them.

Care of rubber catheters

1. Clean immediately after use, with cold water.
2. Drop into boiling water for 2 minutes.
3. Wash with soap and tepid water, rinse thoroughly, dry, and put away.

Care of glass utensils

1. Clean immediately after use, with cold water.
2. Place in cold water and boil for 2 minutes after water comes to a boil.
3. Dry thoroughly and put away.

Care and Arrangement of Flowers[1]

Flowers are a "thrill of encouragement and a will to live" to the weary hearts of the sick and as such should be accorded the same respectful attention as medicines and treatments.

These beautiful messages of hopefulness and love are often made short lived and unsightly by improper treatment, and their proper mission entirely defeated. Nothing but a few minutes of interested attention and some simple rules are necessary for the care of hospital flowers.

Points to be remembered

1. Keep all flowers out of direct drafts.
2. The freshest flowers will soon languish in vases too small for their length of stem, and only half filled with water.
3. Flowers crowded too tightly not only droop quickly, but lose half their beauty by this loss of natural grace and charming pose.
4. Always use deep, roomy bowls or vases, with water enough to cover the stems a little more than half their length.
5. In case a bowl sufficiently deep is not procurable, dampen a newspaper heavily and wrap around the stems. Insert the flowers, paper and all, into the small bowl filled with water. The papers will keep the stems moist and the flowers fresh.
6. In the case of arranged baskets of cut flowers, be sure that the receptacle contains sufficient water.
7. Water potted plants daily, and change the water on cut flowers daily.
8. It will prolong the life of cut flowers to clip a little from the stems every day.
9. Flowers should be removed from patient's room at night.

Care of flower room

1. Wash shelves and sink with soap and water.
2. Leave room in order after arranging flowers.

Care of the Linen Room

Aim

1. To have the linen as conveniently placed as possible and in order at all times.

Necessary articles

Linen.
Blankets.
Pillows.
Rubber sheets.

---

[1] Irene V. Kelley, *Textbook of Nursing Technique*, p. 27.

Procedure
1. Linen:
   a. Wipe the shelves in the linen room with a cloth wrung from warm, soapy water.
   b. Have a definite place for each piece of linen.
   c. Place all pieces uniformly on the shelves so that the fold of linen will be to the front.
2. Blankets:
   a. Fold from top to bottom and then fold in half again.
   b. Then fold ends to center with stripes on the inside.
   c. Place in space provided for them so that the fold of blankets will be to the front.
3. Rubber sheets:
   a. Roll on wooden pole provided for them.
4. Pillows:
   a. Pile neatly on the shelf.

LESSON IV
The Serving of Food to the Sick

Aim
1. To nourish the sick.

General instructions
1. Follow the doctor's orders.
2. Have the tray clean, neatly set, conveniently arranged, and as attractive as possible.
3. Serve food *promptly*.
4. Serve hot foods hot on hot dishes.
    a. See that steam table is turned on 15 minutes before serving food, and that the dishes to be warmed are put in warming oven.
    b. If tray is taken to patient while a treatment is being given, take food back to kitchen and see that food is kept hot.
    c. Serve convalescing patients first and helpless patients last.
5. Serve cold foods cold on cold dishes.
6. Avoid serving greasy, over- or under-done food.
7. Do not serve too many varieties at any one time, for example, liquid diet: tea and soup.
8. Keep the patient in a cheerful frame of mind.
9. Use diplomacy rather than force in getting patient to take food.
10. Do not hurry the patient.
11. Do not serve the dishes too well filled; a second serving is preferable.
12. Encourage the patient to masticate the food well.
13. See that the patient is in a comfortable position before being served.
14. Before serving a tray, remove medicine glasses, emesis basins, etc., from the bedside table and place the tray in a convenient position for the patient to reach.
15. Cut meat for patient if he is unable to do so himself.
16. Serve food to very sick patients often, and in small quantities.
17. Consider the preferences of the patient in serving and seasoning food.
18. In carrying liquids of any kind to a patient in a cup or glass, always carry on small tray or saucer.

Feeding a patient who is in a reclining position
1. Protect patient's gown and bed with a napkin or towel. Dry mouth with napkin as necessary.
2. In giving liquids pour a small quantity into a cup, raise the head slightly by slipping the arm and hand under the pillow. If the head is raised too far forward, it makes it difficult for the patient to swallow.
3. Drinking tubes are preferable to lifting the head unless the

patient is too weak to draw fluid through a tube. Always clean a tube at once after it has been used.
4. Never use a glass tube in feeding a delirious patient. A dessert spoon may be used in feeding a delirious or unconscious patient. Pass the spoon back in the mouth, pressing the tongue gently with the spoon, and the food will generally be swallowed. Carry but a small amount of food in the spoon and do not feed too fast. A rubber ear syringe or medicine dropper can be used to feed a patient if other means fail.

Care of Serving Room or Diet Kitchen

The tray rack
1. Is metal, painted or enameled.
2. To be cleaned weekly with soap and water by maid.
3. The rack is marked in sections.

Trays
1. Keep trays in their respective sections.
2. Bring the tray from the ward as soon as the patient has finished eating.
3. Handle dishes carefully to avoid unnecessary breakage and noise.
4. Keep the door of the kitchen closed.
5. Put remnants of food in garbage can and stack dishes on the maid's table.
6. Wipe tray, spread with fresh napkins, and return to its place on rack.
7. Wipe salt and pepper shakers, fill, and place on tray.
8. If sugar is contaminated, empty sugar bowl and wash. Refill bowl and place on tray. Sugar thus used may be collected for cooking.
9. Weekly care:
   a. Stack trays on maid's table to be washed with soap and water.
   b. Empty and wash salt and pepper shakers.
   c. Empty and wash sugar bowls.

Care of tray of isolated patient
1. Complete isolation:
   a. These trays are not brought into the kitchen.
   b. Carry dishes to and from the patient's room on a second tray protected by napkins.
   c. If it is necessary to put the tray down, put it on the rack.
   d. Carry the dishes back on the second tray protected by napkins.
   e. Remnants of food are put in paper.
   f. Roll the paper up and put it into the waste can in the service room.

g. Put liquids in hopper and flush.
h. Drop dishes into pan of water ready for boiling. Boil 10 minutes.
i. Sterilizer can be used if provided in special isolation department.
j. Dishes are then cared for by the maid.
2. 24 hour isolation:
a. Bring the tray into the kitchen, clean, and care for dishes as in complete isolation.

Nourishment dishes
1. The nurse is responsible for dishes and utensils used for nourishment.
2. Wash as used.
3. If necessary to leave for a short time, cover with cold water.

Glass drinking tubes
1. Do not let fluids dry in them.
2. Rinse in cold water immediately after use.
3. Then wash with water and soap, using special brush.
4. Boil in 1 dr. of sodium bicarbonate to 1 qt. of water.

Tea towels
1. Ordered from laundry at regular intervals by the maid.
2. Kept in drawer of the cabinet.
3. Keep only enough for use.
4. Used towels are hung neatly on the rack.
5. Do not use for any other purposes than drying dishes.

Gas stove
1. Cleaned by maid.
2. The nurse should be very careful to remove any food that spills over.

Kitchen utensils
1. Should be cleaned well after use.
2. Boil teapots in soda solution (1 lb. sal soda to 1 gallon water).
3. After cooking cocoa or milk, rinse in cold water and clean.

Diet kitchen chart
1. Object: An easy, accessible form for showing names of all patients in the ward and the kind of diet they are to be given.
2. Articles necessary:
a. Small white cards.
b. Small colored cards.
c. Small diet chart.
3. Method of indicating diets:
Red..............general diet.
Pink.............. light diet.
Yellow...........semisolid diet.

Green.............liquid diet.
Blue.............. special diet.
White.............name of patient.
Place white card with name of the patient under correct colored card. Patient's name on the tray with adhesive or on colored card of diet.

Nurses are not permitted to eat in diet kitchens:
1. Food belongs to the patients.
2. Dishes have been used by sick people.
3. Time belongs to the patients.

Food is not to be distributed to anyone but patients.

Duties of Senior Nurse on Diets

1. Make out slip showing number of patients, kinds of diets, supplies on hand, and give head nurse before 8 A. M.
2. Supplies ordered one morning are delivered the next.
3. Check list when supplies are received.
4. Responsible for:
   a. Putting supplies in ice box.
   b. Cancellation of trays for patients (breakfast, lunch, and dinner).
   c. Giving test meals, barium meals, Sippy diets.
5. Measure fluids on trays in accordance with intake list. Special attention to those limited.
6. Responsible for:
   a. Feeding helpless patients.
   b. Boiling isolated trays.
   c. Condition of cupboards and ice box.
   d. Keeping up lists.
      (1) Breakage list; check breakage with list every Tuesday. (See form below.) Be sure box is *clean* and lined with paper before sent to office.
      (2) Keep up nourishment list; try to please patient whenever possible.

Med. III
Breakage List
August 10, 1925

DATE	ARTICLE	NAME
August 12, 1925	1 glass	E. Thompson
August 13, 1925	1 plate	Mr. Olson (patient)

......................(Head Nurse)

......................(Sr. on Diets)

LESSON V
BED-MAKING
The Making of an Open and Closed Bed

Aims

1. Comfort of the patient.
   a. Tight foundation.
   b. Not too tight over feet.
2. Sanitation—bedding not to touch floor or uniform.
3. Economy of time, of linen, of energy.
4. Neat appearance while working and when finished.

Necessary articles

2 large sheets.
1 draw sheet.
1 spread
2 pillow cases.
2 pillows (1 small pillow and pillow case in addition in private rooms).
1 rubber draw sheet.
2 wool blankets.
1 mattress pad.

Procedure

1. Place chair at foot of bed.
2. Place clean bedding on the chair in the order to be used.
3. Remove cases from pillows, if necessary, and place in hamper.
4. Place pillows flat on the chair.
5. Loosen bedding all around.
6. Fold spread top to bottom and then in half and place in hamper or over back of chair.
7. Fold blankets, top sheet, cotton draw sheet, rubber draw sheet, bottom sheet, and mattress pad in the same manner.
8. Turn mattress end to end.
9. Put on the under sheet with wide hem at the head, allowing 8 inches to tuck under at the head of mattress. (Unfold all linen on the bed and do not shake.)
10. Tuck under tight and smooth at the head.
11. Fold the corner and make an angle of 45 degrees (envelope fold).
12. Tuck under at the foot and fold the corner as at the head.
13. Begin at the middle, tuck under rest of sheet.
14. Place rubber draw sheet across center of bed, upper edge 8 inches from head of mattress.
15. Cover with cotton draw sheet, tucking 2 inches over the edge of rubber draw sheet.
16. Tuck in both draw sheets.

17. Walk around the bed, turn back the draw sheets, and repeat steps 10-16.
18. Put on upper sheet (wrong side up) with seam of wide hem even with head of mattress.
19. Tuck in the foot, making envelope corner.
20. Place first blanket, upper edge 8 inches from head of bed. Fold lower edge over even with edge of mattress and tuck under at side.
21. Put on second blanket, upper edge 8 inches from head of bed. Tuck in at foot making square corner and tucking under at side.
22. If it is an empty bed, or "closed bed," turn top sheet down over edge of blankets, making a fold of 12 inches. Turn hem under making a finished fold of 8 inches.
23. Put on spread, right side up, top edge even with head of mattress.
24. If an occupied bed, turn the spread over the edge of blankets and the sheet down over the spread. Turn under hem and make finished fold of 8 inches.
25. Walk around bed, turn loose bedding up on bed. Finish as other side.
26. Place pillows flat, open end of case away from the door.
27. If open bed make a fold underneath on seam of pillow case, and place with fold under patient's shoulder.
28. If closed bed, place pillow with fold underneath on seam of pillow at head of bed.
29. Remove soiled linen, replace chair.

LESSON VI

BED-MAKING, Continued

The Making of an Operative or Ether Bed

Aim

1. Convenience in caring for the patient.
2. Warmth for the patient.
3. Comfort for the patient.
4. Protection for the bed.

Necessary articles

1 spread.	1 woolen blanket or bath blanket.
2 mattress pads.	Rubber protector 12 inches wide and
2 large sheets.	long enough to tuck in on both sides
2 wool blankets.	at head of bed.
2 cotton draw sheets.	2 safety pins.
1 rubber draw sheet.	Mouth wipes (cellu wipes or paper nap-
2 pillows.	kins cut in fourths).
2 pillow slips.	Cornucopia or paper bag.
Roller bandage.	2 kidney basins.
Pencil and paper.	3 hot water bottles or bed warmer—
Three tongue blades.	temperature of water 150° F.

Procedure

1. Strip bed.
2. Turn mattress.
3. Make foundation bed.
4. Place rubber protector at head of bed.
5. Cover with cotton draw sheet folded lengthwise and fold surplus under protector at the bottom.
6. Tuck ends under mattress.
7. Place blanket on bed even with top of mattress. Fold back corners at foot to meet in center.
8. Fold top down 8 inches from top of mattress.
9. Fold blanket over on open side even with edge of mattress.
10. Place top covers on bed. Do not tuck in. Finish top in usual way.
11. Make 8 inch fold of all covers even with foot of mattress.
12. Make 8 inch fold on side to be opened.
13. Fold towel over top edge of the upper bedding.
14. Tie the pillow to the head of the bed with a bandage.
15. Place hot water bottles under the blanket at the top, middle, and bottom of bed. (Never leave hot water bottles next to patient unless temperature of water conforms to regulation.)
16. Pin paper bag or cornucopia to cotton draw sheet at upper edge of bed.
17. Pin mouth wipes to cotton draw sheet at upper edge of bed.

18. Cover stand with half of towel, wrong side toward table, and place on it kidney basins, tongue blades, pencil and paper, and cover with the other half of towel.
19. When patient returns:
    a. Remove hot water bottles.
    b. Fold bedding and cotton blanket to opposite side of bed.
    c. Place patient in bed.
    d. Cover with bedding.
    e. Wrap patient well in blanket, tucking around the shoulders.
    f. Adjust towel under chin.
    g. Tuck in bedding at foot and corners in usual manner.

LESSON VII
MISCELLANEOUS PROCEDURES
To Give a Bed Pan or Urinal

Aim

1. To place pan in proper position.

Procedure

1. Warm the pan with hot water, dry, and carry covered to the bed.
2. Place on chair and screen patient.
3. Flex the knees.
4. Draw gown back.
5. Hang bed-pan cover over rail of bed.
6. Put hand under coccyx and place pan in position.
7. Leave toilet paper within patient's reach.
8. When taking a bed pan to a male patient, also take a urinal.

To give a urinal

1. Cover and carry to bedside.
2. Lift the bedclothes at the side of the bed and place the urinal within the reach of the patient's hand.
3. Cover the urinal and remove to service room.

To Remove a Bed Pan

Aim

1. To leave patient and bed clean upon removal.

Procedure

1. If patient is unable to care for himself, wind several thicknesses of paper around hand, cleanse and dry the rectum.
2. Place hand as before and with the other draw the pan down and out.
3. If necessary bring basin and water and cleanse and dry buttocks with toilet paper.
4. Leave body clean and dry.
5. Adjust the bedclothes.
6. Always cover bed pan when removing it to the service room.
7. Ventilate ward.

To clean bed pan

1. Examine contents.
2. Rinse pan first in cold water, then with bed-pan brush clean thoroughly and scald.

To Fill a Hot Water Bottle

Necessary articles

Hot water bottle.   Pitcher.
Cover.   Bath thermometer.

General instructions

1. Be sure that the bottle is in good condition.
2. Always take the temperature of the water with a bath thermometer. *Do not test temperature in any other way.*
3. Expel the air and be sure that the bag is not too heavy.

Procedure

1. Test the bottle to see that it does not leak by putting on the cover and squeezing the bag to see if any air escapes.
2. Fill the bottle ½ full of water at 120°.
3. Expel the air by folding bottle in half and pressing water to neck of the bottle.
4. Screw in cap.
5. Test for leaks by turning bottle upside down.
6. Cover and apply to affected area.

Care of the bag after use

1. Empty the bottle.
2. Wash with soap and water and hang up to dry.
3. When dry, fill with air by drawing the sides apart.
4. Screw in top and put away.
5. If not to be used for a long time powder inside.
6. In case of infection, use same procedure as for ice bag.

To Fill an Ice Cap

General instructions

1. Be sure that the cap is in good condition.
2. Be sure that the metal cover fits and has a rubber washer.
3. Expel the air and be sure the cap is not too heavy.
4. Do not puncture the cap with sharp pieces of ice.
5. Always replace the cover to prevent the cover and washer being lost.

Articles necessary

Ice cap.
Ice.
Cover for the ice cap.
Small pitcher for warm water.

Procedure

1. Break the ice into pieces about the size of a walnut.
2. Pour warm water over the ice to take off the edges.
3. Test the cap to see that it does not leak by putting on the cover and squeezing the bag to see if any air escapes.
4. Fill with ice ⅓ to ½ full.
5. Expel the air from the bag by drawing the top and bottom apart and squeezing the sides together as much as possible.
6. Screw on the cap and wipe dry.
7. Cover and apply to affected area.

8. If it is to be applied to a part where as little weight as possible is desired, suspend it from a cradle or from rolls made of pillows.

Care of cap after use

1. Empty the cap.
2. Wash with water and soap.
3. Dry inside and out.
4. Inflate with air by drawing out the sides.
5. Screw on the cap and put it away.
6. If not to be used for a long time, powder inside.
7. If infected, immerse in 1 per cent liquor cresolis for 20 minutes. Clean and dry as above.

The Application of Binders

Aim

1. To keep applications and surgical dressings in place.
2. To make compression.
3. To afford support and comfort to the patient.

General instructions

Carelessly and inefficiently applied binders are worse than none.

Kinds of binders

1. Scultetus or many-tailed binders.
2. Straight binders.
3. T-binders.
4. Hernia or male T-binders.
5. Breast binders.

Procedure

1. Scultetus:
   a. Fanfold binder half way and place under the patient in such a way that center of binder will come to center of back.
   b. Draw out on other side.
   c. Apply from below toward chest folding strips alternately and obliquely, being careful to arrange smoothly and snugly.
   d. Pin binder, placing pins lengthwise. Use as many pins as are necessary to hold binder in place.
2. Straight binder:
   a. Fanfold binder and place under patient in such a way that center of binder will come to center of back.
   b. Draw out on other side.
   c. Fold ends of binder until it just meets over the largest part of the body.
   d. Pin binder down center.
   e. Pin a dart down each side so that binder will fit patient.
3. T-binders for perineum:
   a. Place around patient's waist.

b. Bring the strip attached to back of straight band that encircles the waist, up over perineum to hold dressings in place.

c. Pin to binder in front being careful that pad is in place and strap not too tight.

4. Hernia binder adjusted same as T-binder.

5. Breast binder:

a. Fanfold binder and place under patient in such a way that center of binder will come to center of back.

b. Draw out on other side.

c. Place breasts in proper position away from axillae.

d. Pin from lower edge of binder to upper edge.

e. Pin straps over shoulder.

f. Pin a dart down each side if necessary for fitting of binder.

To Change the Gown

The hospital gown

1. Loosen soiled gown.

2. Draw off one sleeve, slip clean gown underneath soiled one, covering chest.

3. Put on sleeve by crushing together so that patient's hand can be grasped through opening.

4. Draw over arm and shoulder.

5. Remove other sleeve.

6. Finish putting on the gown and tie the strings.

The long, closed gown

1. To remove soiled gown:

a. Loosen about neck.

b. Flex the patient's knees.

c. Bring lower part of gown up close to buttocks.

d. Slip hand underneath back just below the waist.

e. Raise the buttocks at the same time with the other hand hand slipping gown to waist.

f. Raise head and shoulders as in changing pillows, with other hand draw gown about the shoulders.

g. Remove one sleeve, then raise head, and slip gown off over head; remove other sleeve.

To put on gown

1. Crush together back of gown.

2. Put on one sleeve, crush as with hospital gown.

3. Raise head and slip gown over head.

4. Slip other arm into gown.

5. Raise head and shoulders, draw gown to waist.

6. With knees flexed raise body by placing hand under back below waist.

7. With other hand draw gown below hips then down over legs and ankles.

To Replace Upper Bedclothes with a Bath Blanket

Procedure

1. Fold bath blanket crosswise.
2. Fold open edges back to fold, one on each side.
3. Place folded blanket across chest of patient with the open edge toward the head of the bed.
4. Have the patient hold the lower open edge or tuck it securely around his shoulders.
5. Face the foot of the bed and grasp the other open edge between the fourth and fifth fingers.
6. Grasp the upper covers between the thumb and other two fingers.
7. Fanfold the covers to the foot of the bed.

LESSON VIII

PREPARATION OF THE PATIENT FOR THE NIGHT

(Time of Care Depending on Hospital Routine)

Aim

    1. To make the patient comfortable.

Types of patients

    1. Patients who are up:
        a. See that they are kept clean.
        b. See that they use their own towels, soap, etc.
        c. Things that patient is not permitted to get himself will be brought to him.
    2. Bed patients:
        a. The remainder of this lesson applies to bed patients.

Necessary articles

    Basin of warm water.
    Toilet basket.
    Kidney basin.
    Cup with mouth wash.
    Drinking tube.
    Necessary linen.

Procedure

    1. Place screen around bed if in ward. If in a room, place screen before door.
    2. Arrange articles ready for use.
    3. Lower back rest, remove pillows and all unnecessary articles.
    4. Fanfold top bedding down and replace with bath blanket.
    5. Care of the face and hands:
        a. Protect bedding with face towel.
        b. Wash and dry face.
        c. Place towel on the bed under the arm and hand.
        d. Put basin on the towel and place the hands in the water.
        e. Use the brush if necessary.
        f. Dry the hands, remove the basin and towel.
    6. Care of the teeth:
        a. Place towel and kidney basin under the patient's chin.
        b. Put tooth paste on the brush and pour water over it. If the patient is unable to brush his teeth, gums, and tongue, the nurse will do it for him.
        c. Follow brushing by rinsing of mouth with mouth wash.
        d. Remove kidney basin and towel.
    7. Care of the back:
        a. Remove the gown and place on chair to air.
        b. Remove binders.
        c. Turn patient on side.

d. Expose the back.
e. Spread the bath towel on the bed lengthwise with one edge next to the patient's back.
f. Wash the neck and back with soap and water.
g. Be sure that the hips are clean.
h. Put alcohol in palm of hand and rub back until dry. Rub with long downward strokes and a rotary motion rotating outward from the spine. Work evenly and smoothly, with a firm, gentle, and effective touch. Hands must be smooth, warm, and dry. Avoid jerking or jarring the patient.
i. Dust back lightly with powder.
j. Fold the towel and replace one sleeve of gown.
k. Brush out crumbs and tighten foundation bed. Put on a fresh draw sheet if necessary.
l. Turn patient toward you and finish cleansing and rubbing of back, shoulders, and hips.
m. Finish putting on gown.
n. Walk around bed and complete brushing out crumbs and tightening of foundation bed.
8. Remove bath blanket, pull up upper bedclothes, and straighten.
9. See that patient has an extra blanket and fresh water.
10. Attend to any other requests of patient.
11. Remove screen.
12. Leave room or ward in order.
13. Care of articles used:
a. Clean, replace, and put in proper places.

LESSON IX

FOR THE COMFORT OF THE PATIENT

Aim
1. To make and keep the patient comfortable.

General instructions
1. Never discuss a patient's condition in his presence, even though he may be unconscious.
2. Never discuss a patient's condition with another patient.
3. Satisfy the questions of patients, whenever possible, in accordance with good judgment and common sense.
4. Never go out of a room without leaving it in a better condition and more agreeable for the patient and with a happier atmosphere than when you entered.
5. When possible complete a piece of work, leaving it in a finished condition, before starting another piece of work.
6. Sources of discomfort:
   a. Bad ventilation and bright light in eyes.
   b. Noise, loud voices, whispering, hard heels, squeaky shoes, leaking faucets, banging doors, squeaking hinges.
   c. Letting the patient remain in one position too long.
   d. Extremes of temperature.
   e. Lack of cleanliness.
   f. Weight and pressure on sensitive parts.
   g. Wrinkled bedding.

To Keep a Patient from Slipping Down in Bed

Articles needed
Hair pillow and bandaging.
Rubber pillow case.
Large sheet.

Method No. I
1. Cover pillow with rubber case, roll, and fasten with bandage.
2. Fold the sheet diagonally and beginning at the folded corners roll the pillow in it.
3. Flex the knees and slip the roll under the knees.
4. Place the open part of the roll away from the patient's body.
5. Fasten to the head of the bed with the corners of the sheet.

Method No. II
1. Using one large sheet, fold diagonally 10-12 inches wide.
2. Slip below the patient's feet and bring one end to either side of the bed and tie to the springs.

To Arrange Pillows

Methods
1. To relieve tension on muscles of the abdomen, flex the knees, and support by means of a rubber-covered pillow.
2. To relieve the tension on the muscles of the back, slip a small pillow under the small of the back.
3. To support the patient on the side:
   a. Place a pillow beside the patient for support of abdomen.
   b. Turn the patient on his side.
   c. Turn the pillow under the patient's head diagonally, fitting it in close to the neck and shoulders.
   d. Place a third pillow next to the patient's back.
   e. Place a small pillow between the patient's flexed knees.

To Move a Patient in Bed

Moving a patient from one side of the bed to the other
1. Flex patient's knees.
2. Place one arm under patient's neck and shoulders supporting patient's head on upper arm.
3. Place the other arm well under patient's back on the opposite side.
4. Draw upper part of body toward edge of bed.
5. Slip one hand under lower part of back and the other on the opposite side under the hips.
6. Draw the lower part of the body toward the edge of the bed.

Turning a patient on his side
1. Stand at the side of the bed toward which the patient is to be turned.
2. Place the arms over the patient's body and slip one hand under the shoulders and the other under the hip.
3. Gently but firmly roll the patient toward you. Make sure he is lying squarely and comfortably on shoulder and hip. The lower leg should be extended and the upper flexed and resting on the bed.
4. If the patient is to be left on the side, the hips should be moved toward the center of the bed.
5. A pillow may be placed lengthwise at patient's back, tucked close up for support.

Turning a patient with a draw sheet.
1. Patient must be near the center or farther side of bed.
2. Grasp the ends of the draw sheet from the far side of the bed and turn the patient toward you.
3. Support patient as previously instructed.

LESSON X

FOR THE COMFORT OF THE PATIENT, Continued

To Lift a Patient From a Stretcher to a Bed

Aim
1. To lift a patient with the least possible discomfort and strain to patient and to nurses.

Necessary articles
Stretcher with patient covered with blanket.
Open bed.

Procedure
1. Have a bed ready to receive patient.
2. Bring the stretcher to the bed, placing head of stretcher at foot of bed at an angle of 135°.
3. Three nurses come to the same side of stretcher (inner angle).
4. First nurse places hands under patient's head and shoulders.
5. Second nurse places one arm under back and the other under buttocks.
6. Third nurse places one arm under upper part of legs and the other under the lower part of legs.
7. Lift patient in unison, holding him forward and resting on nurses' chests.
8. Together walk out of step along stretcher and bed to proper place.
9. Lower patient to bed gradually.
10. First nurse—cover patient and remove stretcher blanket.
11. Second and third nurses—remove stretcher.

To Lift a Patient

General instructions
1. In moving or readjusting a patient, always have all articles ready, warm, dry, and in a convenient place.
2. Fold all bed and body clothes so that the patient will never be exposed and yet will not be hampered by them.
3. The nurse's feet should be placed far apart and well supported on the floor.
4. Her knees should be flexed and then straightened as the patient is lifted.
5. Always flex the body at the hips; the body does not flex at the small of the back and by attempting to bend the back and lift, the muscles of the back are unnecessarily strained.
6. When two persons are carrying a patient, always step in unison.
7. Do not lift the patient alone if he is heavy or unmanageable.
8. When lifting a patient, reach beyond the center of weight.

9. Give best support to heaviest parts of body.
10. When lifting, support the framework of the body and do not pull on the muscles and skin nor allow the hands to slip.

To lift a helpless patient up in bed

1. Flex the patient's knees.
2. Nurse A slips one arm under patient's head and shoulders and one arm under small of patient's back.
3. Nurse B slips one arm just below Nurse A's and one under the thigh.
4. Nurse A gives signal to lift and both lift at once.

To lift a patient up in bed when patient is able to assist

1. Flex patient's knees.
2. Patient puts hands on either of nurse's shoulders, or grasps head of bed.
3. Nurse puts one arm under patient's shoulder and one under patient's thighs.
4. Have patient lift himself by his arms and support himself and push with his feet.

To lift an injured arm or leg

1. Never grasp an injured limb alone or change the position of a limb by grasping the fingers or toes.
2. Never place the hands directly under the injured parts.
3. When lifting an injured part, place both hands beneath the injured limb on either side of the injury and raise slowly and gently.
4. In cases of fracture before application of splint, the hand should make slight tension when lifting so that the ends of the broken bones are kept apart.

To Carry a Patient with One Helper

The four-handed seat

Practical only when patient can assist, as in injury to lower extremities.

1. Place chair in proper position with relation to bed.
2. Have patient sit on side of bed or in chair.
3. Slip hands under hips grasping each other's wrists forming a four-handed seat. A grasps left wrist with right hand. B does same. A, with left hand, grasps B's right wrist and B, with left wrist, grasps A's right wrist.
4. The patient sits in the chair thus formed with an arm around the shoulders of each helper. A gives word when to lift, carry, and lower to chair.

The three-handed chair

1. Take position as before. Make seat of three hands. B grasps left wrists with right hand, A's right wrist with left. A

grasps B's wrist with her right.   A's left arm is free to support the patient.

The two-handed chair

1. The same except that the seat is formed of A's right hand and B's left hand, each grasping the other's wrist.
2. A's left arm and B's right are free to support the patient.

To carry patient sitting in chair

1. The chair should be a strong straight-back one:
   a. A and B each grasp chair, one hand at back and other grasping front chair leg.
   b. Lift and carry at word from A.

To Help a Patient Walk

1. The patient's arm is drawn across the helper's shoulders and the body partially supported by grasping the wrist of that arm.   The helper puts his other arm around the patient's waist.
2. The helper's arm is put across the patient's shoulder with the hand in the opposite axilla.   With the other hand the helper grasps the upper arm nearest him.

LESSON XI

FOR THE COMFORT OF THE PATIENT, Continued

The Use of Mechanical Devices

Aim

1. To make a patient comfortable by means of various mechanical devices.

Kinds of devices

1. Back rest.
2. Bed cradle.
3. Knee rolls.
4. Rubber rings.
5. Cotton rolls.
7. Substitutes.
8. Splints.
9. Fracture beds.
10. Orthopedic beds.
11. Electric bakers and cone lights.
12. Electric pads.

Procedure with various devices

1. Back rest:
   a. Aim:
      (1) To get the patient up on a back rest with the least possible exertion and to make him comfortable in that position.
   b. Necessary articles:
      Two or more pillows, large and small. Back rest.
   c. To get a patient up on the back rest:
      (1) Place extra pillow on table at right side of bed.
      (2) Slip arm under pillows and move head and shoulders of patient with pillows over toward right side of bed. Fold bedding to patient's waist line.
      (3) Take back rest around to farther side of bed and set it up in position (about an angle of 60 degrees) placing it as near center of bed as possible.
      (4) Return to right side of bed.
      (5) Slip left arm under patient's head and right shoulder. Support patient with the right arm in front of patient's chest and over the left shoulder and let him lean over that arm, resting head on nurse's shoulder if weak.
      (6) With left hand remove pillows from bed and place on table.
      (7) Reach across and draw back rest into place.
      (8) Place first pillow well down at foot of back rest.

(9) Place second pillow above it.

(10) If more pillows are used, make patient comfortable by filling in hollow places, etc.

(11) Lean patient back on pillows.

Note: Two nurses are necessary where the patient is too ill to sit up without support.

2. Bed cradles are frames made of wire, iron, wood, or wicker in the shape of three or more half hoops resting on flat runners and held in position by cross-bars. They are used to prevent the bedclothes from resting on tender parts:

   a. Place cradle over injured part.

   b. Arrange bedding neatly over frame.

   c. Keep part warm by using extra blankets over frame.

3. Knee rolls:

   a. Cover a pillow with a rubber pillow slip and make in a roll.

   b. Flex patient's knees and slip roll under. This relieves abdominal tension and helps patient to relax muscles.

4. Rubber rings to relieve pressure on bony prominences:

   a. Inflate the ring by covering the valve with a layer of gauze and blowing it about half full of air.

   b. Cover with a pillow slip.

   c. Slip under patient as a pillow. The valve should be at one side, not under the patient.

5. Cotton rolls (called the "doughnut") to relieve pressure on bony prominences:

   a. Cut a square of cotton.

   b. Roll it diagonally and make it into a ring of the desired size.

   c. Wrap it firmly with gauze bandaging.

   d. Slip under any bony prominence or between the patient's knees or ankles. It is sometimes used under patient's ears or heels.

   e. If patient is restless fasten in place by bandage.

6. Sandbags are heavy ticking bags of different weights and sizes filled with sand; they are used to keep a part immobile or as a support or foundation for other appliances:

   a. Cover sandbag with a towel.

   b. If used to avoid foot drop and act as a support, place the sandbag at patient's feet and tuck a pillow over each side making an elevation so that bedclothes do not touch toes.

7. Substitutes for mechanical devices:

   a. Barrel staves cut in two and covered with gauze may be used as a bed cradle.

   b. A box with the ends removed serves the same purpose.

c. A wide board placed at the foot of the bed may be used to elevate bedclothes.

8. A splint is an appliance of wood, metal, plaster, hard rubber, stiff felt, or cardboard used in the treatment of accidents or diseases of the bones and joints and for the correction of deformities to secure local immobility of the part affected or to support an injured part.

   a. General instructions:
     (1) Choose a splint that will extend slightly beyond the joint above and below the seat of injury, and a trifle wider than the part to which it is applied.
     (2) Pad the splint well to prevent chafing. Absorbent cotton and bandages are often used.
     (3) Apply the splint firmly (not too tight to interfere with circulation).

   b. Necessary articles:
     (1) Splint.
     (2) Bandage.
     (3) Cotton.
     (4) Adhesive.

   c. Procedure:
     (1) If practical, wash the area before applying the splint.
     (2) If strapping is to be used, shave the area.
     (3) If abrasions are present, they are dressed.
     (4) Muslin bandage and adhesive are usually used to secure the splint.

   d. After care:
     (1) Wash the skin with soap and water when splint is removed.
     (2) Use alcohol to cleanse any abrasions.

9. Fracture beds:
   a. Aim:
     (1) To keep mattress from sagging.
     (2) To prevent mattress from moving.
   b. Necessary articles:
     Large perforated board the size of the springs.
   c. Procedure:
     (1) The board or boards are placed under the mattress.
     (2) The bed is made in the usual manner.

10. Orthopedic beds:
   a. Aim:
     (1) To keep the covers from resting on the injured limb.
   b. Necessary articles:
     Straight board, cradle, or knee roll.

c. Procedure:
   (1) Make a foundation bed.
   (2) Place cradle over limb, or use knee roll or straight board at the foot of the bed. (The limb may be covered with a bath blanket, if desired.)
   (3) Put the top linen on the bed, being very certain that it is on straight.
   (4) Pull the bottom edge of the bedding down over the foot board, cradle, or knee roll, so that it hangs about four inches below the mattress.
   (5) Pull the sheet and blankets tightly across the foot of the bed, and tuck each under the mattress separately, making as neat a corner as possible.
   (6) Do the same to the spread, only pin it through the covers at corner of the mattress to keep it drawn taut over the foot board.
   (7) Pull the spread down in a straight line, making a square corner.
   (8) Pin this corner to the part of the spread which is drawn over the foot of the bed, thus making it more secure and neat. (Put the safety pins in so that that they will not show.)

11. Electric bakers and cone lights:
   a. Aim:
      (1) To relieve pain and stiffness in inflammatory joints.
      (2) To stimulate the absorption of exudates around joints.
      (3) To relax tissue and increase the blood supply in phlebitis.
      (4) To abort or to hasten the action in carbunculosis.
      (5) To relieve pain in fractures.
      (6) To produce hyperemia in infected wounds.
   b. Duration of treatment:
      (1) Continuous for 24 hours.
   c. Necessary articles:
      Cone light:
         1. Flannel covering.
         2. Safety pins.
         3. Cradle.
      Electric baker.
   d. Cone light:
      (1) If the cone light is ordered over the leg it will not stand upright long, therefore it is necessary to use a cradle.
      (2) Pin the flannel cover around the cone light, covering the edges well.

(3) Place the light over the desired area, and fasten the cone light to the cradle to stabilize it.
(4) Turn on the electricity.
(5) Do not cover the cone light with the bedding.
e. Electric baker:
    (1) Place over area.
    (2) Turn on electricity.
    (3) Replace covers.
f. Record:
    (1) Hour and treatment.
    (2) Location and duration of treatment.
12. Electric pads:
  a. General instructions:
    (1) Examine the pad to see if the insulating material is intact.
    (2) It is not wise to leave the pad "on high" for any great length of time.
    (3) Do not allow the pad to get wet.
    (4) There are 3 switches, low, medium, and high.
    (5) Do not put pins into the pad.
  b. Aim:
    (1) To supply a constant heat.
  c. Procedure:
    (1) Cover the pad with a pillow case or canton flannel cover.
    (2) Attach the plug to a socket.
    (3) Fold or wrap the pad in place.
    (4) Start current on low and increase as needed.
    (5) Shut off the current when through.
    (6) Return pad to school office when not in use.

Fowler's Position

Aim

1. For the comfort of the patient in some medical diseases.
2. To localize infection in the pelvic cavity, promote drainage, and relieve strain on the abdominal muscles and sutures after surgical operations.

Procedure

1. Sit the patient upright in bed, properly supported with back rest and pillows to prevent him from slipping down.
2. Flex the knees and support from underneath by pillows or other support, such as a hammock made by folding a sheet diagonally and tying it to the head of the bed.
Note: For further material on Fowler's position see Harmer, *Principles and Practice of Nursing* (1926 ed.), Chap. XXXIII, p. 577.

LESSON XII
MORNING CARE OF A BED PATIENT INCLUDING MAKING THE BED

Aim
1. Comfort.
2. Cleanliness.
3. Neatness.

Necessary articles
Linen as needed.
Toilet basket.
Wash basin with warm water.
Mouth-wash cup.
Kidney basin.

Procedure
1. Screen patient.
2. Care for mouth and teeth.
3. Place chair at side of bed with clean linen piled in order of use.
4. Loosen bedding all around.
5. Fold spread top to bottom and then in half and place in hamper or over back of chair.
6. Fold top blanket in the same manner.
7. Place bath blanket over patient and remove second blanket and top sheet. Fold like the spread.
8. Remove extra pillows from bed.
9. Remove gown.
10. Lift patient's head and remove pillows.
11. Turn patient on side, face away from you.
12. Examine the patient's back.
13. Wash back with soap and water and rub with alcohol and dust with powder.
14. To change linen:
    a. Roll the draw sheet close to patient.
    b. Roll the rubber sheet close to patient.
    c. Roll the under sheet close to patient.
    d. Straighten the mattress pad.
    e. Pull on clean under sheet, fanfolding the surplus at center and tuck in as for foundation bed.
    f. Draw rubber draw sheet into place, being sure that rubber is regulation distance from the top of the mattress.
    g. Put on clean cotton draw sheet, fanfolding the surplus at center.
    h. Fold cotton draw sheet two inches over top of rubber sheet, and tuck both in at the side.

    i. Replace one sleeve of gown.

    j. Turn patient toward you and finish putting on gown.

    k. Walk around the bed.

    l. Roll cotton draw sheet and remove, pulling clean sheet into place.

    m. Fold back cotton and rubber draw sheets.

    n. Roll under sheet and remove, pulling clean sheet into place.

    o. Straighten mattress pad.

    p. Finish foundation bed and pull up mattress.

15. To make bed without change of linen:

    a. Brush free from crumbs and roll draw sheet close to patient.

    b. Brush free from crumbs and roll rubber draw sheet close to patient.

    c. Brush free from crumbs and roll under sheet close to patient.

    d. Straighten mattress pad.

    e. Straighten and tuck in lower sheet.

    f. Straighten rubber sheet, being sure that sheet is regulation distance from head of mattress.

    g. Straighten cotton draw sheet, folding 2 inches under rubber sheet at the top, and tucking both in at the side.

    h. Put on sleeve of gown.

    i. Turn patient toward you and finish putting on gown.

    j. Walk around the bed.

    k. Repeat steps a-g, and pull up mattress.

16. Turn patient on back.

17. Replace pillows.

18. Replace covers, making a finished fold of 8 inches of sheet over spread.

19. Put towel under the head and comb the hair. Do not neglect to do this.

20. Change pillows:

    a. To remove:

      (1) Slip one arm under head, with hand under far shoulder blade, raise patient slightly.

      (2) With free hand remove pillow by drawing it out from the opposite side of the bed, then placing it on the side of the bed, remove arm from under head.

    b. To replace:

      (1) Place pillow at far side of bed.

      (2) Support patient as above.

      (3) With free hand draw pillow under the head.

      (4) Avoid arranging pillows exactly on top of each other under a patient's head. Endeavor to fit the curve of the neck and shoulders.

LESSON XIII

To Change a Mattress

Aim

1. To change mattress with patient in bed.

Necessary articles

Fresh mattress standing on an obtuse angle from foot of bed (right side).

Procedure

(Two nurses necessary: Nurse A at right of patient, Nurse B at left.)

1. Loosen all covers at head, sides, and foot of bed.
2. Remove top bedding except one blanket and sheet in routine way.
3. Remove pillows, replace by small one if necessary for comfort of patient.
4. Fold upper sheet and blanket over patient to meet in center, folding ends under his feet.
5. Fold upper corners of bottom sheet diagonally toward patient, folding center of upper portion over pillow.
6. Roll sides of lower sheet up to patient's body and tie the ends of the rolls over the patient's feet.
7. A moves the patient to right side of bed by drawing the head and shoulders over gently, then the body, pulling on roll of lower sheets.
8. B pulls mattress to left side of bed until half the wire springs is exposed, rolling up edge of mattress slightly and supporting against her body.
9. A places fresh mattress on exposed springs till it touches the other mattress in the middle. She supports slightly turned edge against her body.
10. A draws patient on to the fresh mattress by drawing over gently, the head and shoulders, then the body, pulling on the roll of lower sheets.
11. B removes used mattress from left side of bed and stands it against the table.
12. B draws fresh mattress into position.
13. B may be dismissed at this point and removes used mattress.
14. A makes up left side of bed with fresh sheets, turns patient to left side of bed, finishing the bed in the usual manner and removing soiled linen.

To Turn a Mattress with the Patient in Bed

Aim

1. To turn the mattress with the patient in bed.

Necessary articles
3 large pillows (including the two on the bed).
1 small pillow.

Procedure
(Two nurses necessary: Nurse A at the right of patient, Nurse B at the left.)
1. Loosen all covers at head, sides, and foot of bed.
2. Remove top bedding except one blanket and sheet in routine way.
3. Remove pillows, replace by small one if necessary for comfort of patient.
4. Fold upper sheet and blanket over patient to meet in center, folding ends under his feet.
5. Fold upper corners of bottom sheet diagonally toward patient, folding center of portion over pillow.
6. Roll sides of lower sheet up to patient's body and tie the ends of the rolls over the patient's feet.
7. A moves the patient to right side of bed by drawing the head and shoulders over gently, then the body, pulling on roll of lower sheets.
8. B pulls mattress to left side of bed until half the wire springs are exposed, rolling up edge of mattress slightly and supporting against her body.
9. B supports the mattress, rolling its edge against her slightly while A places the three large pillows lengthwise on exposed springs.
10. A draws patient on to the pillows by drawing head and shoulders over gently, then the body, pulling on roll of lower sheets.
11. B turns the mattress from top to bottom.
12. A and B lift patient as before from pillows on to the mattress.
13. A removes the pillows and places them on bedside table while B supports the mattress.
14. Draw mattress into proper position on the spring.

LESSON XIV

To Make an Ambulance Bed

Aim

1. To arrange bed in such a way that patient can be put into it easily.

Necessary articles

2 bath blankets.
Rubber mackintosh.
3 hot water bottles.

Procedure

1. Remove pillows.
2. Fold covers to side as for ether bed.
3. Place rubber mackintosh covered with two bath blankets on foundation bed, tucking far side under roll of covers.
4. Place three hot water bottles between bath blankets, as on ether bed.
5. Roll top covers back into place as for ether bed.
6. Pull head of bed away from the wall.
7. Place table and chairs in such a place that they will not be in the way of the stretcher.
8. When patient arrives:
   a. Roll back covers and top bath blanket.
   b. Remove hot water bottles.
   c. Place patient in bed and cover.

To Undress a Patient in Bed

1. Fanfold covers to foot of bed.
2. Remove shoes.
3. Remove clothing from upper part of body.
4. Remove as many articles as possible at one time.
5. Place clothing on back of chair.
6. Put on gown.
7. Remove clothing from lower part of body.
8. When garments cannot be removed whole, rip the seams rather than cut them.
9. To remove tight-fitting shirts, remove as closed night gown.
10. If a portion of the body is injured, remove the clothing from the uninjured side first.

To Dress a Patient in Bed

1. Have all clothing warm and conveniently placed in the order of use.
2. If the garment is closed, make a roll of the hem of the garment to the neck, draw on the sleeves, slip the roll over the head and beneath the shoulders.

3. If the clothing opens all the way down, draw on the sleeve on the side away from you.
4. Turn patient toward you, pull garment well up on the shoulder, and tuck the rest of the garment closely under patient's back.
5. Turn the patient on his back and slightly to the opposite side. Draw the garment beneath the body, slip on second sleeve and adjust. If there is an injury, put the sleeve on the injured side first.
6. To put on stocking, turn the leg of the stocking back over the foot; draw on the foot and then draw up the stocking over the leg.

LESSON XV
ADMISSION AND DISCHARGE OF PATIENTS
Admission of Patients
University Hospital

Aim

1. Make the patient feel at home.
2. Promote the welfare of the patient.

Lesson

1. In the history of nursing, at first the Christian leaders had people come to their homes, where they were sheltered and cared for. The word "hospital" is derived from the word "hostess."
2. Patients are brought to the hospital by ambulance, wheel chair, or on foot.
3. Care of patient begins the moment he enters the ward.
4. Do not meet the patient with the words, "Oh, dear! Here's another case," or with a look of indifference.
5. Do not give the appearance of being in a hurry.

In the office

1. Patient presents application signed by physician and accepted by superintendent of the hospital.
2. The patient's name and address, and the address of the nearest relative are entered opposite the first vacant number in the ledger.
3. The patient is asked to deposit with the clerk any valuables: money, papers, or jewelry. A receipt is sent to the ward with the application blank.
4. Assignment is made to ward and service.
5. The bedside card is filled out, and with the application blank, sent with the patient to the ward.
6. If the patient comes in the ambulance or is unable to go to the desk, the assignment is made and the patient is taken directly to the ward.
7. The social history is taken in the business office.

Routine care in the ward

1. Make patient comfortable.
2. Notify supervisor on the floor.
3. Notify resident and ward physician by telephone.
4. Secure made up chart.
5. Take T. P. R. and record.
6. Fill out temperature and bedside record.
7. Fill out yellow admission sheet.
8. Record name and hospital number on defecation chart under correct service. Record last name first.

9. Record last name on diet chart, light diet unless contraindicated.
10. Record name on census slip with time of admission and service.
11. On surgical service place colored card with bedside card in holder at head of bed.
     Colors: Red—Dr. Law
               Blue—Dr. Ritchie
               Orange—Dr. Wright
               Green—Dr. Burch
12. Admission bath:
    All patients to have tub bath and shampoo except:
    a. Ambulance cases.
    b. Patients having a temperature below 95° or above 100°. These are to have a bed bath.
13. Note general condition and strength of patient:
    a. Physical—disease.
    b. Mental—fear, worry, anxiety over family at home, strangeness, homesickness. This differs in adults and children. Disease may be affected by admission: exposure in coming to the hospital may cause chill and relapse in pneumonia cases; excitement in heart cases; fatigue in cases weakened by sickness.
    c. Strive to prevent or lessen disturbances of patient upon admission. Observe when undressing and bathing the patient the following:
       (1) General appearance.
       (2) Abnormalities.
       (3) Pediculi.
       (4) Fat or thin.
       (5) Edema or loss of flesh (local baggy and wrinkled appearance of skin).
       (6) Poorly or well nourished.
       (7) Rash—evidence of scratching.
       (8) Signs of discharging wounds or ulcers.
       (9) Abrasions or bruises.
       (10) Swelling, growths.
       (11) Loss of motion.
       (12) Loss of special senses.
       (13) Chart all observations and report to head nurse.
14. If emergency or obstetrical case, send specimen of urine to laboratory.
15. List and put away clothes per directions.
16. The ward physician shall take nose and throat cultures immediately after admission of all patients.
17. All patients to be put to bed for 24 hours or until there is a report on nose and throat cultures.
18. Upon admission of any patient who cannot speak for himself,

e.g., a baby, foreigner, unconscious person, etc., the nurse in charge shall detain any person who accompanied the patient to the hospital until the ward physician comes to see him.

How to make a patient feel at home

Shield patient from common causes of annoyance.
1. Do not expose unnecessarily, use screens.
2. Adjust light and ventilation for patient's comfort.
3. Fulfill patient's requests at once.
4. Find out all you can about his likes and dislikes.
5. Never discuss patient's condition in his presence or with his family or friends.
6. Never whisper.
7. Be cordial and firm in meeting patient's friends.
8. Orient patient to surroundings and hospital rules.
   Examples: tell him where bathroom is, what meal hours are, when visiting hours are, etc.
9. Observe patient as a person. Characteristics.
10. Use tact.

Safeguarding the hospital; routine on admission

1. Isolate patient to safeguard other patients from infections and to prevent epidemics.
2. Belongings of patient must be carefully put in safe keeping.
3. Hospital record must be accurate in case of court cases.
4. Accurate charting is the nurse's responsibility and must be authentic.
5. This hospital is a state institution, therefore great care must be taken not to bring harmful publicity.
6. Watch chart carefully to make sure that nearest relative's address and telephone number have been included in social history. It may be necessary to notify someone in a hurry in case of serious illness or death, therefore, ask patient or visitors for names, addresses, and telephone numbers of relatives or friends living in this city or nearby.

Discharge of Patients

University Hospital

1. Discharge blank must be filled out and signed by physician on staff. Ask physicians to complete admission sheet, diagnosis, result, and signature.
2. If patient goes without discharge, he or she must sign own release, or it must be signed by relative or person responsible for the patient. Explain the meaning of the slip to the patient or one responsible and have the slip signed in the presence of a witness. Always notify the interne and ask him to see the patient before permitting release in this way.
3. Enter the patient's name at once on census slip indicating

time and service. Cross name from defecation list and diet chart.
4. No child under 16 years of age is to be discharged without parent or guardian. Name of guardian to be recorded on admission sheet and on bedside notes.
5. If patient has money or valuables in safe, obtain them before 5 P. M. If the patient is to leave on Sunday, get the money on Saturday, as the safe is not open on Sundays and holidays.

Admission of Patients
N. P. B. A. Hospital

In the receiving department

1. Patient presents a slip signed by a company doctor or his employer. If he has no order, ask him to telephone for it. If from out of town, the patient must see the business manager or a doctor of this hospital.
2. Get out the old records if the patient has been here before.
3. Have the business manager see the private patients about the price of rooms. If the patient is a relative of an employee, indicate relationship.
4. Make up a new chart for the patient and fill in all the blanks properly, making sure that a telephone number is obtained. Get a neighbor's number or a relative's, if necessary.
5. The patient is asked to deposit any valuables, such as money, papers, or jewelry, in the safe. The articles are noted in a receipt book. The patient signs one slip, which is kept in the book; the nurse signs the other slip, which is given to the patient. If the patient is unable to look after the slip, it may be attached to the chart. The valuables are placed in a heavy envelope with the name, room number, date, list of valuables, amount, and the nurse's name written on the outside and taken to the business office to be put in the safe. This envelope may be obtained from the office on week days between 8 A. M. and 5 P. M.
6. The temperature, pulse, and respiration are taken and recorded. Likewise the weight and height.
7. The doctor sees the patient in the receiving department, and writes the orders and diet on a slip of paper and attaches it to the chart and room assignment.
8. The patients receive a shower bath before going to the station. The men are given a gown to wear, which they can use as a shirt under their trousers.
9. A room patient's clothing is taken to the room with the patient. A ward patient's clothing is taken to the locker room, leaving out such things as razor, toothbrush and paste, handkerchiefs, and comb, which the patient would want at his bedside. The patient's name is listed alphabetically with the locker

number back of it; the list of the clothes is recorded after the patient's name under the locker number, thus the patient's name is entered twice. Tags with the patient's name on them are put on all loose articles like hats, overshoes, bags, and the like. If any article is removed from the locker, it is checked with red ink and the nurse's initials.

In the ward

1. The receiving nurse takes the patient to the station.
2. The floor nurse assigns the new patient to his bed, if he is a ward patient.
3. Patient is supplied with fresh towels, wash cloth, soap.
4. He is given a glass of fresh water unless contraindicated.
5. Patient is told about signal lights, location of bathroom, mail chute, about the meal time, privileges of any kind, mail delivery hours, visiting hours, name of the head nurse, or any relevant thing. If there are two patients in the room, or a patient in the next bed, introduce them.
6. Put the patient on diet.
7. Enter his name in the temperature book and on the census slip.

Ambulance cases

1. Patients critically ill are admitted to the station at once, and the receiving room nurse gets the data from an accompanying person.
2. The clothing is taken to the locker room by the floor nurses.

Admission of Patients
Minneapolis General Hospital

Aim

1. To make the patient feel at home.
2. To promote welfare of patient.
3. To promote welfare of hospital.

Patients referred to hospital for admission by

1. One of the four city physicians.
2. Police, in cases of emergency and accidents.
3. Recommendation from Hospital Out-Patient Department.
4. Family physician where financial status indicates free care.
5. (Occasionally) recommendation of social service workers.

Lesson

In the history of nursing, at first the Christian leaders had people come to their homes where they were sheltered and cared for. The word "hospital" is derived from the word "hostess."

1. Patients are brought to the hospital by ambulance, automobile, wheel chair, or on foot.

2. Accident cases are taken to emergency rooms, others to examining rooms, in receiving ward.
3. Routine care in receiving ward:
   a. Personal history taken.
   b. Patient undressed.
   c. Examined by physician.
   d. Patient assigned to the proper service.
   e. List clothing and valuables in presence of patient, and have patient sign envelope. Place clothing, marked, in property room. Place valuables in envelopes in safety drawer in receiving office.
   f. Write patient's name in "Clothes and Valuables Books," and state disposition of property.
   g. Notify station that patient is coming.
   h. Make out chart and take to station with patient, together with service card, census board card, and name card for patient's bed.
4. Care of patient begins the moment he enters ward, and great indeed must be the stress of work that will excuse a failure to give him immediate attention.
5. Put yourself in patient's place. Make patient feel at home by having his first impressions pleasant ones.
6. Routine of admitting a patient to ward:
   a. Call interne when patient is admitted.
   b. Temperature, pulse, and respiration taken and recorded.
   c. Register patient's name and register number in census book.
   d. Register patient's name and register number on census board.
   e. Put name card that came with chart on chart back in chart holder.
   f. Put chart on chart back in chart holder.
   g. Bath—if temperature is less than 100°, tub bath; if more, sponge bath. Respect modesty of patient.
   h. Every new patient admitted between 7 A. M and 10 P. M. is to have a bath after admission to the station. The patients admitted at night are to be assigned by the head nurse to nurses in the ward to be bathed the following day regardless of whether it is in the bath ward or not.

Condition of patient observed
1. Physical—disease.
2. Mental—fear, worry, anxiety over family at home, strangeness, homesickness. This differs in adults and children. Diseases may be affected by admission. Examples:

    a. Exposure in coming to hospital may cause chill and relapse in pneumonia cases.
    b. Excitement in heart cases.
    c. Fatigue in cases weakened by sickness.
3. Strive to prevent or lessen disturbances of patient upon admission. Observe when undressing and bathing patient the following:
    a. General appearence.
    b. Abnormalities.
    c. Pediculi.
    d. Fat or thin.
    e. Edema or loss of flesh (local baggy and wrinkled appearance of skin).
    f. Poorly or well nourished.
    g. Rash—evidence of scratching.
    h. Signs of discharge, wounds or ulcers.
    i. Abrasions or bruises.
    j. Swelling, growths.
    k. Loss of motion.
    l. Loss of special senses.
    m. Chart all observations and report to head nurse, also any previous history volunteered by patient.

How to make a patient feel at home

Shield patient from common causes of annoyance.
1. Do not expose unnecessarily; use screens.
2. Adjust light and ventilation for patient's comfort.
3. Find out all you can about his likes and dislikes.
4. Fulfill patient's requests at once.
5. Never discuss patient's condition on his presence or with his family or friends.
6. Never whisper.
7. Be cordial and firm in meeting patient's friends.
8. Orient patient to surroundings and hospital rules, for example, tell him where bathroom is, meal hours, visiting hours, etc. Orient patient as to treatment.
9. Observe patient as a person—characteristics.
10. Use tact.

Safeguarding the hospital

1. Routine in receiving ward: take history and names of relatives or friends in case of death.
2. Isolate patient to safeguard other patients from infections and to prevent epidemics.
3. Belongings of patients must be carefully put in safe keeping.
4. Hospital records must be accurate in case of court cases.

5. Accurate charting is the nurse's responsibility and must be authentic.
6. This hospital is a city institution, therefore great care must be taken not to bring about harmful publicity.

Admission of Patients
Miller Hospital

1. Fill out temperature sheet per sample chart.
2. Fill out diagnosis sheet, showing:
   a. Name, hospital number, division, hour, date, station, and room number.
   b. At the bottom the name of the doctor in charge of the case and the name of the interne.
3. Fill out the social history sheet and sign name at bottom.
4. Ask patient for all valuables: money, papers, or jewelry, for deposit in the office, for which a receipt will be given. Explain that anything of value kept at the bedside must be at the patient's risk. Do not permit the patient to keep any drugs.
5. Take T. P. R. and record.
6. Give bath always, and shampoo, if necessary. Tub or bed bath to be determined by the patient's condition. Any question concerning bath to be determined by the head nurse.
7. List clothes per sample chart and sign name. For tag list see "Instructions for Listing Clothes." The nurse who undresses and bathes the patient is responsible for his or her clothes and valuables unless special assignment is made by the head nurse. The clothes should be cared for immediately following the patient's care. The same rule applies to the night nurses.
8. Put the name of the patient and the doctor's name in defecation chart.
9. Enter name on census slip per sample chart.
10. Enter name on daily report sheet.
11. Call interne in charge of case.

Discharge of Patients
Miller Hospital

1. Discharge blank must be filled out and signed by physician on staff. Ask physicians to complete diagnosis sheet, diagnosis result, and signature.
2. If patient goes without discharge he or she must sign own release, or it must be signed by relative or person responsible for the patient. Explain the meaning of the slip to the patient or the one responsible and have slip signed in presence of a witness. Always notify the interne and

ask him to see patient before permitting release in this way.
3. Enter the patient's name at once on census slip indicating time and service. Cross name from defecation chart, daily report, and diet chart, and notify diet kitchen to discontinue tray.
4. Call main office to ascertain whether bill has been paid before patient leaves the floor.
5. Secure valuables from the office. Patient to sign in office that they have been obtained.
6. See instructions for listing clothes for care at time of discharge.

Care of Patient's Clothing and Valuables
University Hospital

The nurse's responsibility

The nurse who undresses the patient is responsible for the care of his or her clothes and valuables unless special assignment is made by the supervisor. The clothes should be cared for *at once* following the patient's care, either night or day.

To examine clothes
1. Examine for valuables, money, paper, jewelry, drugs, and tobacco.
2. Note if soiled.
3. Examine for pediculi.

To list clothes
1. Make two complete lists (original and duplicate, using carbon paper).
2. Have the patient sign this list.
3. The nurse listing clothes should sign her name in full in space indicated.
4. The original copy is filed with the chart and duplicate fastened on the clothes bag where it can readily be seen.
5. If there is a suitcase or any outside article, tag and place on shelf in clothes room.
6. Any articles withdrawn from the locker or sent home must be indicated on both lists.
7. Note that list of articles retained at bedside must also be signed by patient and nurse.

To put away clothes
1. Put articles on hanger and cover with bag (striped for men, and white for women).
2. Place shoes and small articles in pockets of bag.
3. Place suitcase or bags properly tagged on shelf.
4. Hang alphabetically (see letters on iron posts).

5. Fasten duplicate list to outside of clothing bag.
6. Place in pocket hats or caps if possible to do so without crushing.

Soiled clothes
1. Have clothes taken home for laundry.
2. Clothes that are not washable will have to be cared for at the patient's expense.

Clothes infected with pediculi
1. Place a clean sheet on the table or on the floor, list cloth-on on this, avoiding contamination of other clothing, furniture, or of the floor.
2. Place all woolen garments, or those that cannot be boiled or sterilized, in a sheet and carry to the attic for sulphur fumigation. List those that may be boiled, wrap in a sheet, and send to the laundry marked "boil."

To secure clothes from locker room when patient is discharged
1. Check off each article with red ink on both lists (original and duplicate).
2. If no article is missing sign name at bottom of both lists underneath signature of patient.
3. Have patient sign both lists when he receives clothes.
4. File original list with chart, and place duplicate list on spindle in the school office.
5. Do not throw waste, etc., on the floor in the clothes room.

Care of valuables
1. Ask the patient for all valuables: money, papers, jewelry, etc.
2. Make a list of all valuables and send to main office for deposit in the safe. Instruct the patient that the hospital will not assume responsibility for loss unless valuables are deposited in the safe.
3. Place receipt with the chart.
4. When the patient is discharged:
   a. Receipt is presented to the main office.
   b. Duplicate receipt in book must be signed by patient or person responsible for him.

Care of Patient's Clothing
Minneapolis General Hospital

On admission of patient to receiving ward
1. Examine clothing. Search every pocket and have witness present.
2. Clothing, valuables, and every personal article must be listed on a large envelope *in the presence* of the patient and signed by the patient and by the nurse.

a. A second witness, head nurse and student nurse or head nurse and orderly if the patient is a male, is necessary when the patient is unconscious.

3. Clothing is placed in a canvas bag properly labeled and taken to the property room. One man, on duty from 8 A. M. to 5 P. M., is in charge of the property room. At other times the property room is locked.

4. Contents of bag are to be checked by man in charge of property room and listed in his record book. Clothes are hung on hangers and placed on racks in systematic order. Soiled clothes are labeled, placed in mesh bags, and sent to the laundry.

5. Money or valuables amounting to $5.00 or over are kept in the safe in the property room. Valuables under $5.00 are placed in original envelope and attached to clothes on the hanger.

6. On the discharge of a patient, the head nurse must send a requisition to the property room for the patient's clothes. Such requisitions must be in at 9 A. M. and 1 P. M. The clothes are delivered to the station. The male patients sign for their own articles. On the women's stations the head nurse assumes the responsibility of signing for the patient's clothing.

Care of Patient's Clothing
Miller Hospital

1. The nurse who undresses and bathes the patient is responsible for the care of his or her clothes unless special assignment is made by the head nurse. The clothes should be cared for at once following the patient's care.

2. Examine clothes for valuables (money, papers, jewelry) and for pediculi.

3. Make out list of clothing, listing each article (giving number if more than one) on the provided space on the social history sheet. The nurse listing the clothes reads the list to the patient, and they both sign their names on the social history sheet, thus signifying that the list is correct. When the patient is discharged the nurse checks off each article on the list. The patient signs on the social history sheet "all clothing received" followed by his signature. If patient has a suitcase or bag indicate articles in it on the social history sheet. All clothing and suitcases are to be labeled with the tag having patient's full name, station, room number, and date; for example:

JOHN A. BROWN,
Adm. 241 B
Dec. 12, 1925.

4. If clothing is infected with pediculi place a clean sheet on table or floor, and list clothing on this, avoiding contamination of other clothing, furniture, or floor. Send the clothing with the exception of rubber, leather, felt goods, or other articles which in the judgment of the head nurse should be omitted, in the sheet to the mattress sterilizer.
5. Explain to the patient that anything of value kept at the bedside must be at his own risk. Make a list of all money, papers, and jewelry, and take to the head nurse who will take them to the main office for deposit. The receipt issued will be placed on chart and given to patient at time of discharge. When money or valuables are to be withdrawn from safe, present receipt at office for them. The duplicate receipt must be signed by the person withdrawing valuables. If patient keeps any valuables at bedside he must sign "kept at own responsibility," followed by his name. Nurse witnesses must also sign.
6. If patient dies, check off each article on the social history sheet and have the person responsible for the clothing sign "clothing received," followed by his name.

LESSON XVI
THE BATH
The Bed Bath

Aim
1. For cleanliness.
2. For comfort of patient.
3. To quiet the nerves.
4. To change the circulation.
5. To stimulate the sweat glands.

General instructions
1. Temperature of room may be higher, but not lower, than 80°.
2. The room should be ventilated, but there should be no draught.
3. Temperature of water, 105-115°F.
4. Avoid unnecessary exposure or chilling.
5. If patient chills or is exhausted after or during bath, give hot drinks, apply external heat, and allow him to rest.
6. Examine patient during bath for rash, swellings, discolorations, pressure sores, discharges, abrasions, and vermin.
7. Chart results of observation.
8. Hold corners of wash cloth so they do not drag.
9. Do not leave soap in the water.
10. Always rinse and dry each part thoroughly. Follow with palm of hand to insure drying.

Necessary articles
Linen for changing bed.
Bath blanket.
Kidney basin.
Mouth-wash cup.
2 bath towels.
2 face towels.
1 wash cloth.
Foot tub or bath basin half full of water 105-110°F.
Pitcher of very hot water.
Toilet articles.

Procedure
1. Arrange articles ready for use.
2. Place screen around bed if in a ward, if in a room, place screen before door.
3. Care for mouth and teeth. (For special care of mouth and teeth, see procedure on "Care of the Mouth and Teeth," pp. 63-64.)

4. Place chair at side of bed with clean linen piled in order of use.
5. Loosen upper bedding all around.
6. Fold spread, top to bottom and then in half, and place in hamper or over back of chair.
7. Fold top blanket in the same manner.
8. Place bath blanket over patient and remove second blanket and top sheet. Fold as the spread was folded.
9. Remove extra pillows, etc., from bed.
10. Remove gown, being careful to keep patient well covered.
11. Lift patient's head and remove pillows.
12. Place one face towel under head, and the other under the chin over bath blanket.
13. Wash face, using soap if desired, and dry.
14. Wash neck and ears and dry.
15. Bathe (always bathe far side first), exposing only the part being bathed, protecting bed with one towel and drying with the other in the following order:
    a. Arms, special attention to the axilla.
    b. Hands, placing in basin of water and using brush if necessary.
    c. Chest, protect with bath towel and bathe chest underneath it.
    d. Abdomen (covering chest with bath towel). Protect edge of bath blanket with the other bath towel (if only one bath towel is used, place face towel over chest and protect edge of bath blanket with bath towel).
    e. Thighs and legs.
    f. Protect bed with bath towel, place tub or basin in position in the following manner:
       Put your arm that is nearest the head of the bed under patient's legs and your hand under his heels. Put your other arm across the tub, grasping it on the far side and move it forward into position while at the same time you raise the feet and legs from the bed.
    g. Allow patient's feet to soak. Patient's finger nails may be cleaned while feet are soaking.
    h. Bathe feet and remove tub in the following manner: Put your arm under the legs the same as when putting them into the tub. Pull the tub toward you and place feet on bath towel.
    i. Change bath water and rinse wash cloth and clean tub while in the service room.
    j. Turn patient on side, face away from nurse, and wash and dry back. Rub with alcohol and powder. (If neces-

sary to give special care to back, bring in articles needed before beginning bath.)

k. While patient is still turned on side, rub bony prominences with alcohol and powder (elbows, knees, hips,
and heels).

l. Turn patient on back, allow him, if able, to complete
bath. Place bath towel and well soaped wash cloth
conveniently for patient to reach.

m. Put on one sleeve of gown. Turn patient on his side
and make one half of foundation bed.

n. Turn patient toward you, complete alcohol and powder
rub, and put on other sleeve of gown.

o. Walk around bed and finish foundation.

p. Turn patient on back, replace pillows and towel under
head.

q. Remove bath water and soiled linen.

r. Comb hair.

s. Complete making of bed.

The Prevention of Bed Sores

Aim

1. To prevent pressure sores and to treat pressure sores.

Prevention

1. Constant vigilance on part of nurse.
2. Protect bony prominences from pressure by use of the
following mechanical devices:
   a. Rubber ring.
   b. "Doughnut."
   c. Cradle.
   d. Back rest.
3. Whenever possible, change position of patient frequently.
4. Keep bed clean, dry, and free from wrinkles.
5. Give special care to the back.
6. Protect skin from splints, casts, and restraints by padding
them with cotton.
7. Exercise care when giving and removing bed pan.

Treatment

1. Report reddened spots and abrasions to supervisor.
2. Record condition of pressure sore with time and method
of dressing.
3. For redness and slight abrasions of the skin:
   a. Wash with soap and tepid water and dry by patting,
   not rubbing.
   b. Apply castor oil, tr. benzoin compound, or alcohol, and
   powder.
   c. For involuntary patients apply zinc or boric acid oint-

ment to abrasion or reddened area and keep free from moisture.
  d. Relieve pressure.
4. For deep pressure sores:
  a. Relieve pressure.
  b. Cleanse with irrigations to prevent pus and gangrene formation.
  c. Apply hot boric acid dressings.
  d. Expose directly to air.
  e. Carry out special orders of attending physician.
5. Medications that are often ordered to be used:
  a. Irrigations:
    (1) Boric acid.
    (2) Normal salt.
  b. Powders:
    (1) Talcum.
    (2) Boric acid.
    (3) Stearate of zinc.
  c. Drugs:
    (1) Balsam of Peru.
    (2) Castor oil.
    (3) Zinc oxide ointment.
    (4) Tr. benzoin compound.
    (5) Boric acid ointment.

To Assist with a Tub Bath

Aim
1. For comfort.
2. For cleanliness.

General instructions
1. Have bathroom temperature not lower than 80°F.
2. In case a patient feels faint when in the tub, let the water out of the tub, lower the head and cover patient with a blanket.
3. Do not try to lift a heavy body out of a tub.
4. Assist patient to avoid slipping in stepping out of tub.
5. Never allow a weak or very sick patient or mental case to take a tub bath unassisted.
6. Never turn on hot water faucet when patient is in the tub.
7. Do not leave a patient in the tub of water longer than 10 minutes, unless special orders to the contrary are given.
8. Orderly will assist male patient.

Necessary articles
Kimona.
Bath blanket.

Gown.
Slippers.
Bath towel.
Wash cloth.
Soap.
Chair at side of tub, spread with bath blanket.
Face towel.

Procedure

1. Prepare room and fill tub half full of water.
2. Take patient to bathroom in wheel chair, if unable to walk.
3. Assist the patient to undress, avoiding exposure.
4. Walk to tub with patient, and, standing directly back of her, loosen and hold up kimona or bath blanket about her until she steps into the tub.
5. A bath towel may be draped around patient's hips to avoid exposure while in the tub.
6. Assist patient in washing back.
7. Observe any abnormalities about body.
8. Assist patient in wiping back before she gets out of tub.
9. Hold blanket up about her while she steps out of tub.
10. Dry thoroughly with bath towel.
11. Carry soap and towels to the bedside table.
12. Rinse and wash tub; leave clean and dry.
13. Leave bathroom in order.

LESSON XVII
CARE OF THE MOUTH AND TEETH
General Care

The care of the mouth for convalescent patients and those not seriously ill is the same as in health; it should be kept clean and moist.

Aim
1. To prevent the mucous membranes from becoming dry and cracked.
2. To prevent the formation of sordes.
3. To keep the teeth in good condition.

Time
1. Daily, with morning and evening care.
2. Patients who are very ill must have the mouth cleansed before and after each feeding in addition to the regular care.

General instructions
1. Always wash your hands before and after cleansing a mouth.
2. Use fresh solution and clean sponges for each cleansing.
3. Never dip sponge in the mouth solution a second time.
4. Do not injure the mucous membrane lining of the mouth.
5. Be sure after giving patient necessary articles that he properly cares for mouth and teeth.

Necessary articles
Emesis basin.
Mouth-wash cup.
Toothbrush.
Towel.

Procedure
1. For patients who are able to brush their teeth:
   a. Give the patient the articles necessary for cleansing the teeth.
   b. The toothbrush is kept in a washable bag at the head of the bed, in a container in stand, or in bathroom.
   c. The patient who is able to go to the bathroom will need only the cup of mouth-wash solution.
   d. At the bedside provide cup of mouth-wash solution and a kidney basin.
   e. Provide the patient with a towel. The one provided for the toilet may be used.
2. Care of the helpless patient:
   a. Arrange articles ready for use.

b. Wash your hands.
c. Place the towel under the patient's chin.
d. Place the kidney basin near the mouth on the towel.
e. Pour some solution over the brush.
f. Have the patient separate the teeth enough to relax the mouth.
g. Place the brush with the bristles toward the cutting edge of the teeth.
h. Then turn with a slow sweeping motion.
i. This cleans and at the same time stimulates the gums as well, and cleans the surfaces of the inter-paroximal spaces of the teeth.
j. Rinse the brush frequently while working.
k. If the patient is at all able, have him place the brush as far back on the tongue as he can without causing gagging and brush forward. The patient stands this better if able to use the brush himself. This cleaning must not be omitted even though it is necessary for the nurse to use the brush.
l. To wash the upper lingual surfaces, place the brush bristles up on the roof of the mouth, rotate the brush down over the gums and teeth surfaces. Continue until every surface is cleaned.
m. To wash the lower lingual surfaces, place bristles on gums and rotate upward.

Special Care of the Mouth and Teeth

When given
1. If patient is very ill.
2. If patient has high fever.
3. The condition of the mouth to determine how often.
4. When there is much sordes in the mouth it should be cleaned before and after nourishment.

Necessary articles
Tray.
Cotton pledgets or dental roll in glass jar or in towel.
Forceps or kuroris.
Mouth-wash solution in cup.
Towel.
Drinking tube.
Glass of water.
Tongue blades.
Applicators with cotton.
Lubricant (cold cream).
Lemon juice and glycerine, equal parts, in medicine glass.
Paper bag.

Procedure

1. Proceed as in using brush except that the surfaces are first cleaned by sponging.
2. Moisten pledget and wash thoroughly all surfaces.
3. Then use brush to clean the teeth.
4. Use both pledget and brush on tongue with tongue extended.
5. Have patient rinse the mouth by drawing some of the solution through the drinking tube or by raising the head and taking from the cup.
6. Rinse and have patient expectorate into basin.
7. Apply lubricant as follows:
   a. If the mouth is parched and dry some lubricant such as an albolene flavored with lemon juice is used. Pure cold cream or boric ointment can be used on the lips.
   b. Glycerine and lemon juice, equal parts, is very good to soften sordes before washing and to keep mucous lining soft.

LESSON XVIII
CARE OF THE HAIR
To Destroy Pediculi

Aim
  1. To destroy pediculi.

General instructions
  1. Avoid letting other patients know.
  2. Do not allow patient up and around ward.

Necessary articles
  Tray.
  Rubber pillow case.
  Tr. larkspur or tr. of staphisagria, oz. 3.
  Equal parts of olive oil and kerosene.
  Triangular bandage.
  Cotton balls.
  Dressing towel.

Procedure on head
  1. Protect pillow with rubber pillow case.
  2. Spread face towel lengthwise on pillow.
  3. Using cotton balls, saturate hair and scalp thoroughly with prescribed solution. Have patient keep eyes closed.
  4. Roll hair on top of patient's head.
  5. Cover with triangular bandage and fasten snugly.
  6. Leave this cap on from 12 to 24 hours.
  7. Remove cap at end of this time and examine hair and scalp.
  8. If nits are present apply hot vinegar in the same manner as prescribed solution.
  9. Leave this cap on 12 to 24 hours.
  10. Remove and give shampoo.
  11. Examine hair and scalp.
  12. Repeat process if necessary.

Procedure on body
  1. Daily bath with soap and water.
  2. Follow by bath of bichloride of mercury solution 1-2000.
  3. If ordered, mercury unguentin 33-1/3 per cent to be applied to hairy parts.
  4. Change linen.
  5. Hairy parts may be shaved, if necessary, with patient's permission.
  6. Care of clothes:
     a. If undressing a patient with pediculi, spread a sheet on the floor and pile all clothing on this. Take care in handling clothes not to scatter pediculi to other beds.

Hot box or fumigate with sulphur all clothes that cannot be laundered. (Obtain permission of supervisor.)
b. Bed linen to be put directly in bag used for isolation and sent to laundry.

To Comb the Hair

Aim
1. For comfort.
2. For cleanliness.
3. For tidiness.

General instructions
1. Examine for pediculi or nits.
2. Avoid pulling.
3. Always wash comb after use on each patient.
4. Comb hair every day after morning and evening care.
5. No patient is considered too ill to have the hair combed.

Procedure
1. Protect pillow with towel.
2. Part hair in middle for two braids.
3. If tangled, wet with alcohol, separate into small sections, and comb, beginning at the ends. Grasp the section being combed with the left hand and comb gently.
4. Braid in two braids in any way comfortable to patient, and fasten ends.
5. Occasionally it is necessary to cut matted hair. This cannot be done until head nurse secures *signed* statement from nearest relative granting permission for cutting.

To Give a Bed Shampoo

Aim
1. To wash the hair without discomfort to the patient and without getting the bed wet.

Necessary articles
Rubber sheet, Kelly pad, or shampoo apron.
2 bath towels.
1 wash cloth.
Small pitcher of warm soap solution.
Foot tub or pail.
Small rubber protector.
1 small pillow.
2 pitchers of water, one 115° and the other 105°.
1 face towel.
Hand brush.

Procedure
1. Carry all articles to bedside.

2. Fanfold top covers to waist.
3. Cover patient with bath blanket.
4. Cover small pillow with rubber protector and bath towel.
5. Place small pillow under shoulders, upper edge even with shoulders.
6. Place patient diagonally across bed with head at front edge of bed.
7. Protect bed with rubber sheet, rolling sides to form a drainage pad, or use Kelly pad or shampoo apron.
8. Place foot tub or pan on chair under drainage pad.
9. Loosen and comb patient's hair.
10. Moisten wash cloth and cover patient's eyes.
11. Protecting the ears with one hand, pour water at a temperature of 105° over the hair. With the tips of the fingers use a circulatory movement over the scalp.
12. Pour soap into the hair and lather. Rinse with clean warm water (gradually cooling it) until scalp and hair are clean.
13. Squeeze water from hair.
14. Remove wash cloth from the eyes.
15. Remove Kelly pad and place in pail or tub.
16. Move patient back into position and place pillow covered with bath towel under head.
17. Dry the hair with bath towel over the pillow.
18. When partially dry, place second bath towel under patient's head.
19. Spread hair out and dry.
20. Comb the hair.

LESSON XIX
Restraining Patients

Aim

1. To prevent patients from injuring themselves.
2. To prevent patients from getting out of bed.

General instructions

1. Never restrain patients unless absolutely necessary. Always have a doctor's order before doing it.
2. Make restraint effectual. Careless restraint is worse than none.
3. Prevent any restraint from becoming too tight.
4. Watch for and prevent chafing and pressure sores. Pad wristlets with gauze or cotton and bandaging.
5. If patient is violent, have enough persons to hold him.
6. Do not fasten one side of body only, fasten one hand and opposite foot.
7. Never fasten hands to head of bed.

Articles used for restraint

1. Side boards.
2. Sheets.
3. Handcuffs, anklets, and straps.
4. Straight jackets.
5. Clove hitch.
6. Restraining sheet.

Procedure

1. Side boards are fastened to sides of bed with straps.
2. Sheets:
   a. Fold two sheets diagonally; place one underneath patient's waist and one over abdomen; twist the ends of the two sheets together, draw through the springs, and tie under the springs.
   b. Fold a sheet lengthwise and place across chest of patient, high up under axillae and low down to feet. Twist ends around bars.
   c. Fold sheet diagonally and place under patient's shoulders, bring ends up under axillae, over shoulders, and under the pillow, twist ends together and tie to bar at the head of the bed. (Restraint of the lower part of the body is usually necessary.)
3. Handcuffs and anklets:
   Should be padded. They are adjustable and they lock with a key. Always keep key in definite place. *Never lose key.* (Restrain hand and opposite foot.)

4. Clove hitch:
With a large triangular bandage or with a small sheet folded diagonally, make two loops forming a figure eight with one end up and the other end down. Put loops together with free ends on inside, pass them over hand or foot, twist ends together and make knot 12 inches from extremity and tie to ends of bedside. If not properly applied, it will either not hold or else will shut off the circulation.

To Get a Helpless Patient up Into a Chair

Aim
1. To get a helpless patient out of bed and into a chair with as little exertion as possible, and to make her comfortable.

Articles needed
Chair with arms.
2 blankets.
2 pillows.
1 small pillow.
3 safety pins.
Patient's kimona, stockings, and slippers.

Procedure
1. Place a chair on the right side of the bed with the back of the chair parallel with the foot of the bed. If a wheel chair is used, see that the footrest is up, and that the wheels are locked.
2. Place blanket in the seat of the chair with the top edge even with the chair arms.
3. Fold the second blanket in half crosswise and lay across the back of the chair.
4. Place one pillow in seat.
5. Place second pillow, open end down, against back of chair, with the little pillow at the top for the patient's head.
6. Take patient's pulse.
7. Draw patient to the front of the bed.
8. Slip on patient's kimona and stockings.
9. Fold bedding to the foot of the bed.
10. Flex the patient's knees.
11. With right arm under patient's head and shoulders, and with left arm under knees, lift the patient up and at the same time around into a sitting position with the feet hanging over the edge of the bed.
12. Steady patient for a few seconds.
13. Put on the slippers.
14. Standing directly in front of the patient with one hand in each axilla, slip patient to her feet and at the same time turn her around with her back to the chair.

15. Seat her gently.
16. Put the food board down in place.
17. Fold the bottom of the blanket up over the patient's feet and the sides of the blanket one over the other.
18. Bring the upper blanket together over the patient's shoulders and fasten at the neck with safety pin. Fasten the lower edges of blanket around the patient's wrist.
19. Strip bed, turn mattress, and make up bed.
20. Note patient's pulse 10 minutes after she has been up and after she has been put back to bed.
21. Reverse process to get patient back to bed.

LESSON XX

THE EXTERNAL DOUCHE

(University, Miller, and N. P. B. A. Hospitals)

Aim

1. To cleanse parts:
   a. After perineorrhaphy, curettage, trachelorrhaphy.
   b. After childbirth and abortion.

Necessary articles

Tray containing:
Jar of sterile cotton balls.
Sterile dressing bowl containing sterile cotton balls in ¼ of 1 per cent liquor cresolis compositus solution (approximately one-half dram to one quart—¼ of 1 per cent solution.
Sterile graduate (500 cc.) covered with sterile towel and containing warm sterile water (test by pouring over back of hand).
Sterile forceps (2) in glass of liquor cresolis compositus solution 5 per cent.
Sterile perineal pads.
Paper bag (jar, newspaper, or kidney basin).
Douche or bed pan.
Bed-pan cover.

Procedure

1. Remove pad, fold together, and place at one side.
2. Place patient on douche or bed pan.
3. After urination:
   a. Fold back upper covers except sheet. Drape thighs with upper sheet.
   b. Test the water on the back of the hand.
   c. Pour the sterile water over the parts slowly.
   d. Using sterile forceps number I, take cotton ball from jar, dry parts carefully, using one cotton ball to each downward stroke. Put soiled cotton balls in paper bag. (One forceps is kept sterile for removing cotton balls from jar. Take second cotton ball with forceps number I and then use forceps number II.)
   e. Remove bed pan and apply new sterile pad. Hold in place with T binder.
4. After bowel movement or if secretions or discharges are present:
   a. Fold back upper covers except sheet. Drape thighs with upper sheet.

b. Using sterile forceps, take cotton ball from cresolis solution.
c. Cleanse parts carefully with downward stroke to rectum.
d. Flush the parts with sterile water and proceed as after urination.
e. Turn patient on her side and dry the buttocks.

Record
1. Hour and treatment.
2. Color and amount of discharge.
3. Any redness, swelling, pus forming around stitches, or cutting around stitches.

LESSON XXI
TEMPERATURE, PULSE, AND RESPIRATION

Aim
1. To obtain actual knowledge of the physical condition of the patient by comparison with normal conditions.
2. To aid in making a true diagnosis or prognosis in disease.

General instructions
1. Observe accurately.
2. Never record a temperature, pulse, or respiration carelessly or inaccurately.
3. Never take the pulse inaccurately.
4. Know the relative value of facts as observed.
5. Be able to describe these conditions accurately.
6. Be sure patient has not had anything cold or hot in mouth before taking mouth temperature.
7. Do not take temperature of an unconscious or delirious patient, or of a patient having difficulty in breathing.
8. Do not take what is called a "pen and ink T. P. R."

Where to take temperature
Mouth, 98.6; axillae, 97.6; or rectum, 99.6, because large blood vessels are near the surface at these points.

When to take temperature
1. q. 4 h.
2. As ordered by attending physician.
3. All patients with temperatures of 100° and above.
4. B. i. d. (when patient has no elevation of temperature).

Articles necessary
Thermometer tray with:
Thermometers (rectal and mouth).
Three glasses with cotton in bottom.
Glass of water.
Glass of bichloride solution 1-1000.
Jar for clean wipes.
Jar for waste wipes.
Vaseline.
Glass with bichloride for rectal thermometer.

Procedure
1. Mouth:
   a. Place thermometer in glass of bichloride solution 1-1000.
   b. Take thermometer from solution and wipe with paper square.
   c. Rinse in water and wipe with paper square.
   d. Shake mercury below 95°.

e. Place end of thermometer containing the mercury under the tongue. (The mouth should be thoroughly clean.)
f. See that lips are closed tightly and that patient breathes through nose only.
g. Leave thermometer in mouth for 2 minutes or more depending on grade of thermometer.
h. Remove, wipe with paper square, read, and replace in bichloride solution.

2. Rectum:
a. Remove thermometer from bichloride solution.
b. Wipe with paper square.
c. Shake down to 95°.
d. Lubricate with vaseline.
e. Turn patient on side or leave on back if more convenient.
f. Insert thermometer slowly, bulb end first, up to 98°.
g. Allow to remain 2 minutes.
h. Remove, wipe with paper square, and read.
i. Replace in bichloride solution.

3. Axilla:
a. Use same technique as for taking by mouth.
b. Remove sleeve of gown.
c. Place end of thermometer containing the mercury in the hollow of axilla.
d. Have patient hold arm down tightly.
e. Leave for 5 minutes.
f. Remove and use the same technique as for mouth.

Care of tray
1. Empty bichloride solution, wash glasses, and refill q. A. M.
2. Empty water glass after each use of tray and leave dry with fresh cotton.
3. Empty and clean jar for waste wipes.
4. Refill jar with clean wipes if necessary.
5. Leave pencil on tray.
6. Change towel under glasses p. r. n.
Note: See Harmer, *Principles and Practice of Nursing* (1926 ed.), Chapters XIII, XIV, XV, for further material on temperature, pulse, and respiration.

LESSON XXII
OBSERVATION, COLLECTION, AND CARE OF
SPECIMENS
Collection and Care of Specimens
University Hospital

Aim
1. To aid in diagnosing disease.

Preparation of specimen bottles
1. Aim:
   a. To have proper receptacles ready for specimens.
   b. To prevent contamination of the specimen.
2. General instructions:
   a. Be sure specimen bottles are clean.
   b. Use no cracked receptacles.
   c. Secure the right kind of receptacle for each kind of specimen.
   d. Specimen bottles supplied from the laboratory.
3. Types of specimen containers:
   a. Urine specimens:
      (1) Morning specimens in 4 oz. bottle with large mouth.
      (2) Twenty-four hour specimens in 1 gallon bottle.
   b. Sputum:
      (1) Sputum cup.
   c. Vomitus:
      (1) Conical glass. A wax-lined pasteboard box can be used.
   d. Stools:
      (1) Wax-lined pasteboard box (ordinary specimens).
4. Method of sterilizing bottles:
   Wash bottles thoroughly and put in sterilizer filled with cold water or fill bottles with hot water and place in boiling sterilizer. Have sufficient water in sterilizer to cover the bottles. If corks are used sterilize at the same time. Boil ten minutes. Use sterile forceps to take out bottles and put in corks, or plug with a sterile cotton ball.

General instructions for collecting specimens
1. Urine (may be collected by voiding and by catheterization):
   a. Routine morning specimen from all new patients first morning in ward.
   b. By special order of doctor.
   c. Emergency surgical cases and obstetrical cases immediately upon admission.
   d. 24 hour specimen:

(1) Note time specimen is to be started, 6 A. M. usually.
(2) Have patient void but do not save the specimen; always begin the collection with an empty bladder.
(3) Label with patient's name, date, 24 hour specimen, hour started, number of floor, hour closed, interne's name, and nurse's initials.
(4) Collect and save in gallon bottle all urine voided during the next 24 hours.
(5) Have patient void at the end of 24 hours (6 A. M.) and add it to the urine collected.
(6) Send entire specimen to laboratory with request blank made out correctly.

e. P. S. P. specimen:
(1) Have patient empty bladder immediately before injection of phenolsulphonephthalein.
(2) Have patient drink two glasses of water.
(3) Collect first specimen exactly one hour and ten minutes after injection.
(4) Collect second specimen exactly one hour from time of first collection.
(5) Send both specimens to laboratory in small bottles with request blanks filled in by doctor.
(6) If patient is unable to void at correct time report to supervisor.
(7) To avoid the test being incorrect caution the patient not to void until told to do so.
(8) Chart: P. S. P. given by Doctor————(in red ink).
A. M. 9:10 Spec. I sent to laboratory.
A. M. 10:10 Spec. II sent to laboratory (in black ink).

f. Mosenthal specimens:
(1) Mosenthal test meal (special diet) given at 8-12-4.
(2) Have patient empty bladder at 8 A. M. Specimen not to be saved.
(3) Prepare six small bottles and one large one.
(4) Collect specimens at 10-12-2-4-6-8, and save all of each specimen and put in separate bottles. Label each with patient's name, hour voided, date, floor, and "Mosenthal."
(5) After the 8 P. M. specimen has been collected save all other voidings until 8 A. M., having patient void at exactly 8 A. M. Save in large bottle and label "Mosenthal test," patient's name, date, floor, and "12 hour specimen 8 P. M.—8 A. M."
(6) If test is repeated next day, collect specimen as for first day.
(7) Keep all specimens in cool place and send to laboratory with request blanks when test is over.

(8) Chart: Mosenthal test (in red ink). Specimens collected every 2 hours from 10 A. M. to 8 P. M., inclusive. at 10-12-2-4-6-8 (in black ink). From 10 P. M. to 8 A. M., inclusive, 12 hour specimen saved.

g. Urine specimens from babies:
(1) Boy babies: test tube, finger of rubber glove, adhesive.
(2) Girl babies: test tube, adhesive square.

2. Sputum:
a. Save A. M. specimen unless otherwise ordered.
b. Have patient expectorate directly into pasteboard sputum box if possible. Put cover on closely and send to laboratory with request blank.

3. Stomach contents:
a. Obtain by saving vomitus or remove contents by aspirating.
b. Send to laboratory in conical glass with request blank.

4. Feces:
a. Transfer defecation from bed pan to specimen box and cover securely.
b. Send to laboratory with request blank.
c. Stools to be examined for parasites are to be sent immediately after passed to laboratory in bed pan. Mark bed pan with number of floor.

Collection and Care of Specimens

N. P. B. A. Hospital

Aim
1. To have the proper receptacle for specimen ready.
2. To prevent contamination of specimen.

General instructions
1. Be sure that the bed pan, the patient, and the specimen bottle are clean. Sterilize the receptacle if it is to be used for the examination of bacteria.
2. Label the bottle correctly in pencil with the patient's name, date, room number, kind of specimen, and nurse's signature. If it is a preoperative specimen write "preoperative" in red ink in the upper left hand corner.
3. Secure the correct container for the specimen:
a. Urine:
(1) Four ounce bottle.
(2) Liter glass jar.
b. Stools:
(1) Wax-lined paper board box.
(2) Bed pan if entire specimen is desired.
c. Sputum:
(1) Sputum cup.

(2) Board of Health bottle.
d. Vomitus or stomach contents:
(1) Enamel dressing basin.
e. Spinal:
(1) 3 bottles properly labeled.
f. Thoracentesis:
(1) Sterile test tube.
g. Vaginal smear:
(1) Glass slides (dry, lay smear side down on paper).
h. Blood chemistry, Wasserman, and throat cultures are taken by technician.
4. Do not use a cracked receptacle.
5. Prevent contamination of specimen.
6. Procure quantity sufficient for examination.
7. Collect specimen at time ordered.
8. Cover specimens immediately after placing them in receptacle.
9. Chart all specimens sent to laboratory.
10. Have orderly take specimens to laboratory before 7 A. M. (The orderly brings the bottles up during the night for the night nurse.)

Procedure
1. Urine:
a. Morning specimens:
(1) Medical department:
(a) For all new patients.
(b) For all patients showing albumin.
(c) For all nephritics.
(d) For all diabetics.
(e) For all chronics, urinalysis once a month.
(f) Doctor usually orders for private patients.
(2) Surgical department:
(a) For all new patients.
(b) For all operatives.
(c) For all postoperatives (2 days).
(d) For all patients showing albumin or sugar.
(3) Obstetrical department:
(a) For all new patients; if not obtained before delivery, wait 5 days.
(b) For all patients having more than a one plus albumin.
b. 24 hour specimen:
(1) Note the time for the specimen to begin (usually 6 A. M.).
(2) Have the patient void at 6 A. M. and destroy the specimen.
(3) Label the specimen jar with the patient's name, room number, date, hour started, and nurse's name.

(4) Collect all urine for the 24 hours; if any is lost, estimate the amount and record it on the slip.

(5) Have the patient void at the end of 24 hours (6 A. M.), add to and close the specimen.

(6) Have the orderly take the specimen to the laboratory before 7 A. M.

(7) Chart: 24 hour specimen to laboratory.

(8) Start another bottle, following the same routine.

c. P. S. P. test:

(1) Have the patient empty his bladder immediately before the injection of 1 cc. ampule of phenolsulphonephthalein into the lumbar muscle.

(2) Give the patient 2 glasses of water to drink.

(3) Collect the first specimen one hour and ten minutes after the injection and label it "No. 1." Collect second specimen one hour after the collection of first specimen and label it "No. 2."

(4) If the patient is unable to void, report it to the doctor.

(5) Send the two specimens in separate bottles to the laboratory.

(6) Chart in red ink: "P. S. P. test" (by doctor, if he does it); in blue ink "specimen to laboratory." In the urine column, chart "specimen to laboratory."

d. Mosenthal specimens:

(1) Give patient special diet 7-12-5, encourage him to eat entire meal, and not to eat or drink anything not ordered.

(2) Instruct patient to void at 8 A. M.; destroy specimen.

(3) Collect specimen at 8-10-12-2-4-6-8; label properly with the hour obtained and keep separately.

(4) Collect all urine in one bottle from 8 P. M. to 8 A. M. and label "12 hour specimen."

(5) Send the specimens to the laboratory.

(6) Chart in red ink: "Mosenthal test"; in black ink: "specimens collected at 8 (for control) -10-12-2-4-6-8, and 12 hr. specimen at 8 A. M."

e. Urine specimens from babies:

(1) Boys: use a test tube, rubber finger cot, and adhesive.

(2) Girls: use a test tube and a square of adhesive (stick the edges of adhesive around the vulva and secure with with strips of adhesive).

2. Stools:

a. Remove a part of the specimen with a tongue blade to a waxed container, label, chart, and send to laboratory.

b. If the specimen is being examined for parasites, take it to the laboratory while warm and notify the technician.

c. If the specimen is being examined for tapeworm, call the technician to the service room to see the specimen.

d. Chart: "specimen to laboratory."

3. Gastric contents:

a. Take the patient to the dressing room for the expression.

b. Collect the specimen in the white enamel dish provided for this purpose (call for this dish at the laboratory later on in the day and return it to the tray).

c. Label the specimen and take to the laboratory.

d. Chart in red ink: "Gastric specimen by Dr. Blank"; in blue ink: "specimen to laboratory" and any other comments if necessary.

4. Sputum:

a. Save the early morning specimen.

b. Collect the specimen in the regulation State Board of Health bottle, having the patient expectorate directly into the bottle.

c. Write the patient's name only on the bottle and send to laboratory.

d. Chart in red ink in the bedside-notes column: "sputum specimen to laboratory."

Collection and Care of Specimens

Minneapolis General Hospital

Aim

1. To aid in diagnosing disease.

Preparation of specimen bottles

1. Aim:

a. To have ready proper receptacles for specimens.

b. To prevent contamination of the specimen.

2. General instructions:

a. Be sure specimen bottles are clean.

b. Use no cracked receptacle.

c. Secure the right kind of receptacle for each kind of specimen.

d. Specimen bottles supplied from laboratory with preservative, toluol and chloroform. Formalin used at General Hospital.

3. Types of specimen containers:

a. Urine specimens:

(1) Morning specimens 6-8 oz. bottle.

(2) Twenty-four hour, 4 quart bottle.

b. Sputum—vomitus:

(1) Wax-lined pasteboard box (ordinary specimen).

c. Stomach contents:

(1.) Glass graduate.
d. Stools:
(1) Wax-lined pasteboard box (ordinary size).

General instructions for collecting specimens

1. Avoid contamination of specimen by having all receptacles clean.
2. Have quantity sufficient for examination.
3. Collect specimens at time ordered.
4. Always label specimen and send to laboratory with laboratory request blank.
5. Avoid confusing specimens.
6. Explanation to patients about saving urine saves many mishaps.
7. Chart all specimens to laboratory.

Types of specimens and method of obtaining

1. Urine (may be collected by voiding and by catheterization):
   a. Routine morning specimen from all new patients first morning in ward.
   b. Preoperative specimens.
   c. By special order of doctor.
   d. Emergency surgical cases and obstetrical cases immediately upon admission.
   e. Twenty-four hour specimens:
      (1) Note time specimen is to be started, usually 6 A. M.
      (2) Have patient void but do not save this specimen; always begin collection with an empty bladder.
      (3) Label 4 qt. bottle with patient's name, date, "24 hour specimen," hour started.
      (4) Collect and save all urine voided in the next 24 hours.
      (5) Have patient void at 24 hours (6 A. M.) and add it to the urine specimen collected.
      (6) Send entire specimen to laboratory with request blank labeled "24 hour specimen."
   f. P. S. P. specimen:
      (1) Have patient empty bladder immediately before injection of P. S. P. (To avoid the test being incorrect, caution the patient not to void until told to do so.)
      (2) Have patient drink two glasses of water.
      (3) Collect first specimen exactly one hour and ten minutes after injection. Save all of specimen in a small bottle and label, "P. S. P. No. I," and hour of collection.
      (4) Collect second specimen exactly one hour from time of first collection. Save all of specimen in a bottle and label, "P. S. P. No. II," and hour of collection.

(5) Send both specimens to laboratory with request blank filled in by doctor.

(6) If patient is unable to void at correct time, report to head nurse.

(7) Chart:

P. S. P. given by doctor, 9:10 Specimen I, sent to laboratory; 10:10 Specimen II, sent to laboratory.

g. Mosenthal test specimens:

(1) Mosenthal test meal (special diet) given at 8-12-6.

(2) Have patient empty bladder at 8 A. M. specimen not to be saved.

(3) Prepare six small bottles and one large one.

(4) Collect specimens at 10-12-2-4-6-8, and save all of each specimen and put in separate bottles. Label each with patient's name, hour voided, and "Mosenthal test."

(5) After 8 P. M. specimen has been collected save all other voidings until 8 P. M., having patient void exactly at 8 A. M. Save in large bottle and label "Mosenthal test," patient's name, and hour voided, "Mosenthal Test 12 hour specimen, 8 P. M.-8 A. M."

(6) If test is repeated next day, collect specimen as for first day.

(7) Keep all specimens in a cool place and send to laboratory with request blank when test is over.

(8) Chart: Mosenthal test, specimens collected at 10-12-2-4-6-8, 8 A. M., 12 hour specimen sent to laboratory.

h. Urine specimens from babies:

(1) Boy babies: test tube, finger of rubber glove, adhesive.

(2) Girl babies: test tube, adhesive square.

2. Sputum:

a. Save A. M. specimen.

b. Have patient expectorate directly into wax-lined pasteboard box, if possible. Put cover on closely and send to laboratory with request blank.

3. Stomach contents:

a. Send to laboratory in glass graduate with request blank.

4. Feces:

a. Transfer defecation from bed pan to specimen box and cover securely.

b. Send to laboratory with request blank.

c. Stools to be examined for parasites are to be sent immediately after passed to laboratory in bed pan.

Collection and Care of Specimens

Miller Hospital

Aim

1. To aid in diagnosing disease.

Preparation of specimen bottles

1. Aim:
   a. To have ready proper receptacles for specimens.
   b. To prevent contamination of the specimen.
2. General instructions:
   a. Be sure specimen bottles are clean.
   b. Use no cracked receptacle.
   c. Secure the right kind of receptacle for each kind of specimen.
   d. Specimen bottles are supplied from the laboratory.
3. Types of specimen containers:
   a. Urine specimens:
      (1) Morning specimens in 4 oz. bottle with large mouth.
      (2) Twenty-four hour in 1 gallon bottle.
   b. Sputum:
      (1) Sputum cup.
   c. Vomitus:
      (1) Conical glass. A wax-lined pasteboard box can be used.
   d. Stools:
      (1) Wax-lined pasteboard box (ordinary specimen).
4. Method of sterilizing bottles:
   a. Wash bottles thoroughly and put in sterilizer filled with cold water or fill bottles with hot water and place in boiling sterilizer to cover them. If corks are used, sterilize at the same time. Boil ten minutes, using sterile forceps to take out bottles and put in corks, or plug with sterile cotton ball.

General instructions for collecting specimens

1. Avoid contamination of specimen by having all receptacles clean.
2. Have quantity sufficient for examination.
3. Collect specimens at time ordered.
4. Always label specimen and send to laboratory with laboratory request blank.
5. Avoid confusing specimens.
6. Explanation to patients about saving urine saves many mishaps.
7. Chart all specimens to laboratory.

Types and method of obtaining

1. Urine (may be collected by voiding and by catheterization):
   a. Routine morning specimen from all new patients first morning on ward.
   b. By special order of doctor.
   c. Emergency surgical cases and obstetrical cases immediately upon admission.
   d. Twenty-four hour specimen:
      (1) Note time specimen is to be started, usually 6 A. M.
      (2) Have patient void but do not save the specimen. Always begin the collection with an empty bladder.

(3) Label with patient's name, date, "24-hour specimen," hour started, number of floor, interne's name.

(4) Collect and save in gallon bottle all urine voided in the next 24 hours.

(5) Have patient void at end of 24 hours, or 6 A. M., and add it to the urine collected.

(6) Send entire specimen to laboratory with request blank labeled "24-hour specimen."

e. P. S. P. specimen:

(1) Have patient empty bladder immediately before injection of P. S. P. To avoid the test being incorrect caution the patient not to void again until told to do so.

(2) Have patient drink two glasses of water.

(3) Collect first specimen exactly one hour and ten minutes after injection. Save all of specimen in a small bottle and label "P. S. P. No. I" and hour of collection.

(4) Collect second specimen exactly one hour from time of first collection, save all the specimen in a bottle and label "P. S. P. No. II" and hour of collection.

(5) Send both specimens to laboratory with request blank filled in by doctor.

(6) If patient is unable to void at correct time, report to head nurse.

(7) Chart: P. S. P. given by doctor.
A. M. 9:10 Spec. I sent to laboratory.
A. M. 10:10 Spec. II sent to laboratory.

f. Mosenthal specimens:

(1) Mosenthal test meal (special diet) given at 8-12-6.

(2) Have patient empty bladder at 8:00 A. M. Specimen not to be saved.

(3) Prepare six small bottles and one large one.

(4) Collect specimens at 10-12-2-4-6-8 and save all of each specimen and put in separate bottles. Label each one with patient's name and hour voided, "Mosenthal test."

(5) After 8 P. M. specimen has been collected save all other voidings until 8 A. M., having patient void exactly at 8 A. M. Save in large bottle and label "Mosenthal test," patient's name, and "12 hour specimen 8 A. M. and 8 P. M."

(6) If test is repeated next day, collect specimen as for first day.

(7) Keep all specimens in cool place and send to laboratory with request blank when test is over.

(8) Chart: Mosenthal test. Specimens collected at 10-12-2-4-6-8 A. M. 12 hour specimen saved.

g. Urine specimens from babies:

(1) Boy babies: test tube, finger of rubber glove, adhesive.

(2) Girl babies: test tube, adhesive square.

2. Sputum:
   a. Save A. M. specimen unless otherwise ordered.
   b. Have patient expectorate directly into pasteboard sputum cup if possible. Put cover on closely and send to laboratory with request blank.

3. Stomach contents:
   a. Obtain by saving vomitus or remove contents by aspirating.
   b. Send to laboratory in conical glass with request blank.

4. Feces:
   a. Transfer defacation from bed pan to specimen box, cover securely.
   b. Send to laboratory with request blank.
   c. Stools to be examined for parasites are to be sent to laboratory in bed pan immediately after passed. Mark bed pan with number of floor and patient's name.

Water and Concentration Test

Miller Hospital

1500 cc. water or tea between 7:35 A. M. and 8:15 A. M.

Collect urine, measure amount and specific gravity of each specimen.

8:30 A. M.
9:00
9:30
10:00
10:30
11:00
11:30
12:00
3:00 P. M.
5:00
7:00
9:00
12:00 Midnight
8:00 A. M.

No other fluids in 24 hours. Dry diet.

LESSON XXIII
CHARTS AND CHARTING
Charting
University Hospital

Aim
1. To aid the physician in arriving at a correct diagnosis.
2. To keep an exact record of a patient's condition and the course of the disease.
3. To keep a record of all medications, treatments, and diet.

General instructions
1. Record and chart accurately, concisely, and neatly.
2. Avoid repetition and use of all unnecessary words and phrases.
3. Do not use chemistry symbols.
4. If abbreviations are used they must be correct, and if there are two words to the name both must be abbreviated.
5. Pay close attention to spelling. A dictionary is kept on the head nurse's desk for the use of students.
6. Refer to sample chart.
7. Join dots on last temperature chart before putting on a new chart.
8. Have dots on temperature chart pinhead size.
9. Draw lines with a ruler.

Procedure
1. Temperature record:
   a. Heading of chart sheet should be filled in correctly and each succeeding sheet likewise. If service of staff doctor or interne has changed, see that correct name is filled in.
   b. Day of month: the chart for each day is to be headed with the month, day, and year in figures, as 3-1-22.
   c. Day in hospital. The day of admission counted as one.
   d. Day of operation counted as 1. This is important for surgeons. Record in red ink under day in hospital.
   e. Day of operation indicated in remarks.
   f. T. P. R.:
      (1) Temperature charted with black ink.
      (2) Pulse charted with red ink.
      (3) Respirations charted with black ink.
      (4) Using scale of black figures at left side of chart, indicate the temperature by a dot (pinhead size) in middle of space. Join succeeding temperature by a straight line. Use ruler.
      (5) Using scale of red figures at left of chart indicate the pulse by a dot as for temperature.
      (6) Respirations recorded in perpendicular figures in column indicated.

(7) A chill is indicated by a dotted line from last temperature to temperature which is taken ½ hour after chill.

(8) The temperature following a sponge bath is indicated by a dotted line from last temperature to temperature which is taken ½ hour after completion of the bath.

(9) Write "admitted at. . . . ." in first temperature column.

(10) When patient is operated on, write "day of operation" along temperature column.

g. Stools and urination:

(1) Stools are indicated by Roman numerals.
Stools and urination of all responsible patients are to be charted by temperature and medicine nurse at 4:00 P. M.

(2) For involuntary and irresponsible patients, stools and urination are charted by the nurse attending them.

(3) Urine is indicated by a check except in cases where the doctor has ordered the urine to be measured.

(4) If the patient has had no stools or urinations during the day or night, indicate by a zero.

(5) Observations concerning the stools and urine are recorded in the remark column.

(6) All operative cases, new mothers, and serious accident cases should have all urine measured for the first 48 hours and longer if necessary. Number of cc. of urine recorded in urine column.

(7) Intake and output required routinely on certain cases and other cases according to doctor's orders. The intake and output are totalled and recorded by the night nurse at 6:00 A. M.

h. Diet:

(1) Chart kind of diet and hour in column designated for diets.

(2) If liquid diet, chart kind and amount, also hour.

i. Standing orders:

(1) Record on the day the order is first carried out.

(2) When the order is discontinued record again and write "discontinued" in red ink.

(3) When a new sheet is put on, all standing orders being given at that time are recorded on the new sheet.

2. Nurse's bedside notes:

a. Heading of chart sheet should be filled in correctly and each succeeding sheet likewise. If service of staff doctor or interne has changed, see that correct name is filled in.

b. Draw a red line across chart to divide the days.

c. In date column, write month, day, and year, as, 3-1-22.

d. Diet—chart kind of diet and hour. If liquid diet, chart kind and amount, also hour.

e. Medication—chart hour, medication, and dosage. If a standing order, chart as follows:
Tr. digitalis m. V t. i. d. 8/12/5. Check hour when given with red ink.
If a single order, chart as follows:
P. M. 8 aspirin gr. V.

f. Treatments:
Taken up under procedures for the various treatments.

g. Remarks are charted in column designated for that purpose:
(1) Each nurse should do the charting for the patients assigned to her.
(2) Chart all observations, treatments, and care of patient.
(3) Avoid the repetition of the word "patient."
(4) Fill in whole line; do not leave blank spaces on chart.
(5) Punctuate and spell correctly.

Charting

N. P. B. A. Hospital

Aim

1. To aid in making a correct diagnosis.
2. To serve as a memorandum for the nurse.
3. To be used as legal record in lawsuits.
4. To be used for compiling statistics and historical records.

General instructions

1. Print record accurately, neatly, and concisely.
2. Write the Christian name of married women, e. g., "Mrs. Mary Smith," not "Mrs. Fred Smith."
3. Write the day of admittance as, July 22, 1928, and each day thereafter in figures as, 7/23/28.
4. Write the day of illness, which is the day of admittance, directly under the date.
5. Write the first postoperative day in red ink after the day of illness, e. g., 7/24/28 3/1 (red ink).
A second postoperative day would be started after the first postoperative day in like manner.
6. Record each treatment, medication, and nourishment directly after it has been given.
7. Avoid repetition and use of all unnecessary words and phrases.
8. Do not use chemistry symbols.
9. Use only the accepted abbreviations as: sol. for solution; spec. for specimen; and lab. for laboratory.
10. Do not abbreviate patient, left, right, or abdomen.
11. Do not erase; draw a line through a mistake and label "recorded by mistake." If a chart is recopied, give the two

sheets to the supervisor, have her verify it, and she will destroy the incorrect one. The initials of the nurse who copies the chart should appear in the upper left corner.

12. Do not chart on the last line of the chart; if there are only a few spaces left start a new sheet for the following day.
13. Do not use ditto marks.
14. Record the following in the bedside notes:
    a. Time:
        (1) For each procedure.
        (2) For going to x-ray.
        (3) For going to operating room.
        (4) For returning from operating room.
        (5) For going to physiotherapy.
        (6) For being transferred, giving the room number.
        (7) For being discharged.
        (8) For certification of death.
    b. Patient's symptoms as:
        (1) Nausea and vomiting.
        (2) Stools and urine.
        (3) Abdominal distension.
        (4) Dyspnea.
        (5) Cheyne-Stokes respiration.
        (6) Cough and expectoration.
        (7) Diet and nourishment.
        (8) Surgical dressings.
        (9) Medications; reason for omittance, if omitted.
        (10) Pain, location of.
        (11) Skin conditions, rashes.
        (12) Menstruation.
        (13) Vaginal douche.
        (14) Irrigations.
        (15) Sleep, restlessness, wakefulness, etc.
        (16) Stupor or coma.
        (17) Delirium, irrational; record some of the incoherent things the patient says.
        (18) Hiccough.
        (19) Convulsions, character and duration.
        (20) Chills, duration and temperature.
        (21) Treatments.
        (22) Visits of consultant physician.
        (23) Intake and output.
15. Record the following in red ink:
    a. Medications.
    b. Voiding before going to surgery and the first postoperative voiding.
    c. Dressings, removal of sutures, packs, and drains.
    d. Removal of radium.

e. Treatments:
(1) Gastric expression with doctor's name.
(2) Gastric lavage with doctor's name.
(3) Duodenal expression with doctor's name.
(4) Spinal puncture with doctor's name.
(5) Myringotomy with doctor's name.
(6) Hypodermoclysis with doctor's name.
(7) Intravenous with doctor's name.
(8) Thoracentesis with doctor's name.
(9) Aspiration with doctor's name.
(10) Paracentesis with doctor's name.
(11) Dressings and examination of wound with doctor's name.
(12) Catheterization and bladder irrigation with doctor's name (male patients).
(13) Tests of any kind like tuberculin, Schick, or Dick, with doctor's name.
(14) Basal metabolism test with technician's name.
(15) Electrocardigraph test.
(16) Catheterization and bladder irrigation with nurse's initials.
(17) Hypodermics with nurse's initials (reason in blue).
(18) External heat, if for therapeutic purpose.
(19) External cold.
(20) Sputum to laboratory; specimen to laboratory.
(21) Enemata, results in blue.
(22) P. S. P. test.
(23) Swabbing of throat.
(24) Irrigations.
(25) Proctoclysis.
(26) Turpentine stupes and fomentations.
(27) Plasters and poultices.
(28) Specimen to laboratory.
16. Record the following in blue ink:
a. All comments on patient's condition and the result of treatments.
b. Weight and height.
c. Defecation.
d. Diets.
e. Visits of consultant physicians.
f. Statement of death with doctor's name.
17. Connect all temperature dots before putting on a new sheet.

Necessary articles

Chart back.
Laboratory sheet, form 37.
Personal history sheet, form 27.
Surgeon's injury sheet, if an accident case, form 101.

Admittance sheet:
   a. N. P. patient, form 20.
   b. Private patient, form 19.
Temperature sheet, form 30.
Chart cover.

Procedure

1. Admittance sheet:
   a. Fill in all the blanks accurately.
   b. Obtain a telephone number, neighbor's if necessary.
   c. Have the signature of the admitting nurse.
2. Temperature sheet:
   a. Fill in the blanks accurately.
   b. Record the temperature in blue ink, opposite the hour recorded in the bedside-notes column, making a dot at correct intersection of lines.
   c. Record the pulse in red ink, making a dot as instructed above.
   d. Record respiration in blue ink, writing the number in the space provided for this purpose.
   e. Write the weight and height in the column between 105-107 degrees.
   f. Record the room number in the upper left hand corner below the day of illness.
   g. Record the admission to the ward, whether the patient walked, came on the stretcher, or in a wheel chair.
   h. Record all subjective symptoms of the patient.
   i. Record all abrasions, scars, contusion, or any abnormalities or objective symptoms noticed about the patient.
   j. Stools and urination:
      (1) Write the word "output" in the first space under "respiration, stools, and urine."
      (2) Indicate the stool by a Roman numeral; if no stools, indicate with a zero.
      (3) Record urine, if measured, by cc.; if not measured, merely check the column if the patient is voiding normally.
      (4) Record the urine of all operatives, new mothers, and serious accident cases for 72 hours.
      (5) Record 24 hour specimens at 6 A. M.
   k. Intake:
      (1) Write the word "intake" in the first space between the temperature columns 97-98.
      (2) Intakes are totalled at 6 A. M. as follows:
            1000 cc. mouth
             200 cc. proctoclysis
            1000 cc. hypodermoclysis
            ————
            2200 cc.

1. Diet:
   (1) Chart the kind and hour each day as 7-12-5.
   (2) Record nourishment 10-2.

Charting

Minneapolis General Hospital

Aim

1. To aid the physician in arriving at a correct diagnosis.
2. To keep an exact record of a patient's condition and the course of the disease.
3. To keep a record of all medications, treatments, and diet.

General instructions

1. Record and chart accurately, concisely, and neatly.
2. All charting between 7 P. M. and 7 A. M. is in red ink with the exception of the temperature line.
3. All charts are started in the receiving ward.

Procedure

1. Heading of chart sheet should be filled in correctly and each succeeding sheet likewise. If service, staff doctor, or interne has changed, see that correct name is filled in.
2. Date—each day is to be headed with the month, day, and year in figures, as, 3-1-22.
3. Day in hospital—day of admission counted as one.
4. Day after operation—draw a line through day of disease. Day after operation counted as 1, this is important for surgeons. Day of operation indicated in remarks.
5. Hour—this column indicates time T. P. R. are recorded.
6. T. P. R.:
   a. Temperature charted with black ink.
   b. Pulse charted with red ink.
   c. Respirations charted with black ink.
   d. Using scale of black figures at left side of chart, indicate the temperature by a dot (pinhead size) in middle of space. Join succeeding temperatures by a straight line. Use ruler if necessary.
   e. Using scale of red figures at left of chart indicate the pulse by a dot as for temperature.
   f. When a new sheet is started make temperature and pulse line continuous from one sheet to the next.
   g. Respirations recorded in perpendicular figures in column indicated.
7. Stools and urination:
   a. Stools are indicated by Roman numerals. Stools and urination of all responsible patients are to be charted by the temperature and medicine nurse at 4 P. M.

b. Involuntary and irresponsible patients' stools are charted by the nurse attending them.

c. Urine is indicated by a check except in cases where the doctor has ordered the urine to be measured.

d. If the patient has had stools or urinations during the day or night indicate by a zero.

e. Observations concerning stools and urine are to be recorded in the remark column.

f. All operatives, new mothers, and serious accident cases should have all urine measured for the first 48 hours and longer if necessary. Number of cc. of urine to be recorded in the urine column.

g. Intake and output required as routine on all:
  (1) Med. A. 1 cases.
  (2) Pneumonia cases.
  (3) Uremia cases.
  (4) Other cases according to the doctor's orders.

h. Intake and output totalled and recorded by night nurse at 7 A. M.

8. Diet:
  a. Chart kind of diet and hour in column designated for diets.
  b. If liquid diet, chart kind and amount, also hour.

9. Remarks are charted in column designated for that purpose.
  a. Each nurse should do the charting for the patients assigned to her.
  b. Chart all observations, treatments, and care of patient.
  c. Avoid repetition of the word "patient."
  d. Fill in whole line. Do not leave blank spaces on chart.
  e. Punctuate and spell correctly.

10. Chart treatments and medicines in column designated for that purpose (taken up under procedure on "Administration of Medecines").

Charting

Miller Hospital

Chart definition

1. A permanent, written record, giving true information concerning a patient as follows:
  a. General condition, including symptoms, objective and subjective.
  b. Amount, frequency, and kind of nourishment taken.
  c. Nature and amount of sleep.
  d. Amount, frequency, and nature of excreta.
  e. Amount, frequency, and kind of medication and treatment.

Aim

1. To provide records:

a. For doctor, hospital protection, for patient's benefit in case of readmission, and for statistics and research.
b. As a record of orders given, received, and carried out or cancelled.
c. As an aid to diagnosis and case history.

History
1. Charts were used in ancient times in the form of parchment and tablets, for the Egyptian kings. These have been unearthed in recent years and some very valuable information has been obtained as to treatment, etc. Tablets of the ancient and lost tribe of the Incas in Peru also show records of quite intelligent treatment given for illness.

Essential points in charts
1. Truth and accuracy.
2. Neatness.
3. Brevity and comprehensiveness.
4. Good judgment of essentials; this comes only with practice and should be constantly kept in mind when charting remarks, etc.
5. Good English, writing, and spelling.

Legal aspect of charting
1. A chart is a legal document. A nurse may be called upon at any time to give evidence or corroborate statements she has made on a chart, if the case should become a legal one.

Varieties of charts
1. Infants' charts.
2. General purpose charts.
3. T. P. R. charts.
4. Weight charts.
5. History charts.
6. Medical charts.
7. Surgical charts.
8. Obstetrical charts.
9. Child charts.

Common faults in charting
1. Inaccuracy.
2. Tendency to become mechanical; avoid such statements as "fair night," "poor night," etc.
3. Failure to chart essentials, i. e., amount of sleep, elimination, nourishment taken, improvement or not.
4. Poor writing and printing, grammar, spelling, etc.
5. Temp. chart dot not of uniform size, not enough care given to making straight lines, etc. Ruler should be used.
6. General carelessness, i. e., omission of record number on each sheet, dating each sheet, use of red and black ink.

7. Neglect in the charting of symptoms, when observed, and treatments, etc., when completed. Doctors come in, in the meantime, read the charts, and find nothing there to give them an idea as to the real condition of the patient.
8. Mistakes made and carelessly rubbed out, in place of reprinting the sheet.
9. Fluid diets not printed carefully enough.
10. The patient's name "as it is written on the admission slip" should be recorded on each sheet of the chart. Be careful of the spelling and do not change the name in any way.
11. Condition of patients in the Maternity Department is not always carefully charted.
   a. Condition of the vaginal sutures.
   b. Condition of breasts during the first five days.
   c. Condition of lochia, whether it is profuse, scanty, odor of, etc.
   d. Condition of the fundus, whether soft or firm, high or low.
   e. Whether baby has nursed or not, and if not, why not.
   f. Specimen of urine; some patients having several and others none at all.

Mechanics of charting
1. Use suitable pens, should be fine, not stub pens.
2. Use good ink, red and black.
3. Use ruler, blotters, chart backs.
4. Use paper as good as can be obtained, otherwise it blots.
5. Use rubber bands to hold charts to backs; otherwise they curl and tear.

Records in red ink
1. All records of major importance (not routine orders) and any that are of importance on any particular case.
2. The following are always recorded in red ink:
   a. All tests:
      (1) Von Pirquet.
      (2) P. S. P.
      (3) Schick.
      (4) Tuberculin.
      (5) Vaccines, etc.
      (6) Blood count.
      (7) Wasserman.
   b. To x-ray.
   c. Spinal puncture.
   d. Gastric expression or lavage.
   e. Aspiration of chest.
   f. Paracentesis.
   g. Test meals (in diet column).
   h. To operating room.

i. For operation (in diet column).

j. 24 hour specimen of urine.

k. Specimen of urine or stool to the laboratory.

l. Total cc's of output and intake (in urine and diet column).

m. Per catheter—L. B.

n. Amount of urine voided before going to operating room.

o. First voiding of urine after the patient has returned from the operating room.

p. All other specimens.

q. Bladder irrigation.

r. Weight of patient.

Order for filing charts

1. Diagnosis sheet.
2. Social history sheet.
3. Yellow history sheet:
   a. History.
   b. Physical.
   c. Notes.
   d. Dental.
4. Laboratory sheet:
   a. Urine.
   b. Blood.
   c. Special.
5. X-ray sheet.
6. Consultation sheet.
7. Operation record.
8. Bedside notes.
9. Postoperative record to go in between bedside notes at the date of operation.
10. Remove all blank sheets before chart is sent in to the office. Name, hospital number, etc., to appear in the space provided at the top of all of the sheets except the diagnosis sheet, which has only the hospital number.

Social history

To be filled out and signed by the nurse admitting the patient. Address and telephone number (if any) of nearest relative to be noted very carefully. *This is very important.*

Clothes should be carefully listed by the nurse. Signature of the patient or the relative to be written at the bottom of the list. The name of the nurse listing the clothes must appear on the line provided above that list. Valuables to be taken care of in the office safe; otherwise the patient assumes responsibility if they are lost.

LESSON XXIV
POSITIONS AND DRAPING FOR EXAMINATIONS AND TREATMENTS

Aim

1. To protect the patient during examination and treatment.
2. For the comfort of the patient while different parts of the body are examined.

General instructions

1. Avoid all unnecessary exposure of the body.
2. Protect the patient from other patients in a ward by the use of screens.
3. Drape so that the outline of the patient's figure will not be discernible.
4. Keep the patient covered until the physician comes.
5. Tell the patient the reason for the examination.
6. If a complete physical examination is to be made replace the covers with a bath blanket.
7. Have all the necessary articles at hand.
8. See that the windows are closed and that the shades are up.

Necessary articles

1. Physical examinations:
   Tray with:
   Wooden tongue depressors.
   Paper bag.
   Face towel.
   Flash light.
   Red and blue pencils.
   Tape measure.
   Safety pins.
   Doctor's towels.
   Applicator with pin.
   Percussion hammer.
   Tuning fork.
   Glass slides.
   Note: If examination of eye, ear, and throat is to be made, additional articles must be provided.
2. Gynecological examination:
   Tray with:
   Large sheet.
   Sterile gloves.
   Sterile perineal pad.
   Paper bag.
   Glove powder.
   Doctor's towels.

Lubricant.
Rubber protector.
Bed-pan cover.

Positions

1. Dorsal:
   a. Patient flat on his back, with one pillow under his head.
   b. Knees separated and slightly flexed.
2. Knee-chest:
   a. Allow one small pillow for head.
   b. Patient rests on his chest and knees; knees slightly separated; face turned on side resting on the pillow; thighs perpendicular; arms free at both sides.
3. Sims:
   a. Patient lies on his left side; right knee flexed and drawn up nearly to the abdomen; left knee slightly flexed; left arm is drawn under the side to back; right arm free in front.
4. Lithotomy:
   a. In bed: patient on back across bed, buttocks slightly beyond the edge of mattress, hips slightly elevated with pillows; knees flexed on abdomen and held in position by a strap or by a folded sheet, passed upward, over one shoulder back of the neck, down over the opposite shoulder, and pinned about the flexed knees.
   b. On examining table: patient in the dorsal position with knees flexed. The feet are placed in stirrups at the foot of the table.
5. Trendelenburg:
   a. Patient lies on back on examining table, thighs and trunk elevated on an incline plane of 45 degrees. Legs bent at the knees down on other side of the plane.
   b. Shoulder supports are used to prevent patient from slipping.

Types of examinations

1. Throat:
   a. Have patient in position so that a strong light, at the examiner's back, can be thrown upon the throat of the patient.
   b. If examiner uses head mirror, have light always in front, either natural or artificial.
   c. Always hold tongue depressor in the middle so that the fingers do not touch the portion that is to go into the patient's mouth.
   d. After a tongue blade has been used, it should never be placed on a chair, bed, or table. Put immediately in a paper bag or pus basin and then put it into the garbage can as soon as possible.

2. Chest:
   a. Up patient:
      (1) Remove all clothing from upper part of the body.
      (2) Place sheet folded diagonally about the shoulders pinning it in front.
      (3) Have the patient sit on a stool or chair so that the front and back are accessible.
      (4) If the doctor examines the front of the chest, fold the sheet back over shoulders, if the back, the sheet is turned around with the opening in the back. Then fold back over the shoulders.
   b. Bed patient:
      (1) Remove all but one pillow.
      (2) Always hold towel between patient's face and doctor's head.
      (3) If patient is able to sit up in bed drape as for up patient.
      (4) If not able to sit up, either remove gown and place a towel over anterior chest, or roll hem of gown up so that it does not interfere with the examination.
      (5) To examine back, turn the patient on his side away from the doctor and drape as for anterior chest, or have patient sit up in bed. Support lower back with pillow. Place towel over posterior chest and gown over anterior chest.
3. Abdomen:
   a. Have patient lie in the dorsal position with the knees flexed to relax the abdominal muscles.
   b. Turn all bedding back to pubes and groins and cover patient with towel or blanket.
   c. Place a towel over the abdomen and at the same time draw up the patient's gown and roll it just above the waist line.
   d. During the examination the towel is removed from the abdomen and placed over the pubes.
4. Lower extremities:
   a. Loosen bedding from the foot of the bed.
   b. Fold the spread and the blanket upward.
   c. Leave the sheet to prevent unnecessary exposure of the extremities.
   d. When both legs are being examined bring the sheet between the thighs.
5. Rectal:
   a. Screen patient.
   b. Fanfold upper bedding to the foot of the bed and at the same time cover patient with an extra sheet.
   c. Place patient in dorsal, knee-chest, or Sims position, usually dorsal with knees flexed.

d. Use sheet diagonally and wrap both feet and legs in each corner.

e. Or have patient flex the knee on the side by which the doctor stands, and turn back corner covers. Put a rubber protector and a bed-pan cover under the buttocks.

f. Open package of gloves and hold the right glove for the doctor to put on. Uncover lubricant.

g. Turn back corner of sheet between knees.

6. Vaginal:

   a. Have external parts scrupulously clean.

   b. Have patient relax as much as possible by taking a series of long deep breaths.

   c. Fanfold the bedding and drap the patient with sheet folded diagonally as for rectal examination.

   d. Assist doctor with glove and lubricant.

   e. Protect patient's modesty and sensibilies by control of speech and facial expression.

Care of articles after use

1. Leave tray clean and equipped for future use.

2. Wash gloves with cold water, then with soap and warm water. Boil 3 minutes. Dry thoroughly on both sides.

Record

1. Hour of examination.

2. By whom performed.

LESSON XXV
ENEMATA

General instructions

1. Do not expose the patient unnecessarily.
2. Protect the bed from excretion and odor.
3. Lubricate the tip and do not use force in inserting it.
4. Do not allow air to enter the intestine.
5. Have temperature of the solution 100-105°.
6. In cases of impacted rectum when it seems necessary to use the finger to break up the contents of the rectum, cover the finger with a finger cot or put on a rubber glove.
7. Allow solution to run slowly.
8. Have the correct solution and the exact amount ordered.
9. Position:
   a. Left side—left lateral.
   b. Dorsal.
   c. Knee-chest.

Cleansing or Evacuating Enemata

Aim

1. To hasten evacuation and to wash out the colon.

Solution used

1. Soap solution. Use ivory or castile soap and make a milky solution.
2. Normal saline solution.

Temperature of solution

1. 100° to 105° F.

Amount

1. About 3 pints.

Necessary articles

Irrigator standard.
Bed pan, bed-pan cover, and toilet paper.
Tray containing the following:
   Bath blanket.
   Irrigating can, with tubing (3 feet) and stopcock.
   Rectal tip or rectal tube in kidney basin.
   Vaseline or oil, square of toilet paper for applying.
   Small rubber protector.
   Dressing towel.

Procedure

1. Carry standard, bed pan, cover, toilet paper, and blanket to bedside.
2. Place bed pan and toilet paper on the chair.

3. Screen the patient.
4. Carry tray covered with dressing towel to bedside.
5. Fanfold cover to foot of bed and replace with bath blanket.
6. Place patient in proper position.
7. Raise the gown.
8. Place the rubber protector covered with bed-pan cover under the patient's buttocks.
9. Hang the irrigating can about two feet above the patient.
10. Connect tip or rectal tube.
11. Expel air and warm tube by permitting solution to flow until the tube is filled with warm solution.
12. Shut off flow and lubricate the tip.
13. Insert tip into rectum and open the stopcock.
14. Give the required amount of solution, close the stopcock, and withdraw tip.
15. Disconnect rectal tube or tip and place in kidney basin.
16. Place the patient on the bed pan and give him the signal light.
17. Leave the patient alone unless his condition contraindicates it.
18. When the solution has been expelled, care for the patient as usual.
19. Ventilate the ward.

Care of articles used
1. Carry tray to the service room.
2. Wash irrigating can and tubing.
3. Dry can and return to the shelf.
4. Dry tubing by stripping and draining and coil with stopcock open.
5. Wash rectal tube or tip in cold water; drop into boiling water for 2 minutes. Wash with soap and warm water, rinse thoroughly, and dry. Put away in dry container.

Record
1. Hour and treatment.
2. Amount and kind of solution used.
3. Character of the return flow.

Carminative Enemata

Aim
1. To relieve distention caused by flatus.

Temperature of solution
1. From 110° to 118° F.

Solutions usually ordered
1. Turpentine, 1 dram, olive oil, 4 ounces.
2. Nobles enema: turpentine, 1 dram, glycerine, 2 ounces, magnesium sulphate, 3 ounces, and water, 4 ounces.

3. Tr. asafetida, 2 drams, and water, 4 to 6 ounces.
4. Milk, 8 ounces, and molasses, 8 ounces.

Necessary articles

Bath blanket.

Bed pan, cover, and toilet paper.

Tray with:

    Large funnel with rectal tube (size 24 lengthened to 18 to 24 inches by tubing and glass connection).

    Kidney basin.

    Small rubber protector.

    Bed-pan cover.

    Basin of water 110° F. Place in this a small pitcher containing solution to be given.

    Vaseline and paper square for applying.

    Dressing towel.

Procedure

1. Carry tray covered with dressing towel to the bedside.
2. Carry other necessary articles to the bedside.
3. Screen the patient.
4. Fanfold covers to the foot of the bed and replace with the bath blanket.
6. Raise the gown.
7. Place the rubber protector covered with bed-pan cover under the patient's buttocks.
8. Lubricate the rectal tube.
9. Expel the air by permitting the solution to flow until the tube is filled.
10. With the funnel in the kidney basin, introduce the tube about five inches.
11. Raise funnel and pour fluid on side of funnel to prevent the forcing of the air in the tube into the colon.
12. Proceed as with a cleansing enema.
13. Give the enema slowly and if the prescribed enema is a small one, encourage the patient to retain it from fifteen to thirty minutes.

Care of articles used

1. Carry the tray to the service room.
2. Thoroughly cleanse and sterilize articles.
3. Put articles away.

Record

1. Hour and treatment.
2. Formula and amount.
3. Length of time retained.
4. Character of the return.
5. Amount of flatus expelled.

Emollient, Sedative, and Stimulating Enemata

Aim

1. Emollient: To soothe the irritated mucous membranes.
2. Sedative: To quiet the patient.
3. Stimulating: To stimulate in cases of shock or collapse.

Prescriptions usually ordered

1. Emollient:
   a. Cornstarch, 1 dram, and cold water, 1½ ounces. Mix to a smooth paste and add 5 ounces of boiling water. Boil one or two minutes and cool to 105° F. If laudanum or opium is prescribed, add to the enema just before giving.
   b. Flaxseed, 30 cc., and cold water, 1 pint. Boil for 10 minutes, strain, and inject while warm.
2. Sedative:
   a. Chloral hydrate. Sodium Bromide. Paraldehyd. Mix medication ordered with six ounces of water.
3. Stimulating:
   a. Strong black coffee, 5 to 6 ounces; give it at a temperature of 115° F.

General instructions for enemata to be retained

1. Keep the patient quiet after giving the enema.
2. Avoid all stimuli, either mental or physical, that might excite peristalsis.
3. Have the rectum and colon free from feces.

Necessary articles for above enemata

Bath blanket.
Bed pan, cover, and toilet paper.
Tray with:
   Large funnel with rectal tube (size 24 lengthened to 18 to 24 inches by tubing and glass connection).
   Kidney basin.
   Small rubber protector.
   Bed-pan cover.
   Basin of water 110° F. Place in this a small pitcher containing solution to be given.
   Vaseline and paper square for applying.
   Dressing towel.

Procedure for above enemata

Same as for carminative enema, with the following exceptions:
1. When all the solution has been given, remove the catheter and make pressure against the anus with the bed-pan cover until the desire to expel the solution has ceased.
2. Make the patient comfortable.

Record

1. Hour and treatment.
2. Formula and amount.
3. Whether retained or expelled.
4. Length of time retained.
5. Patient's reaction to the treatment.

Nutritive and Oil Enemata

Aim

1. Nutritive: To provide nourishment.
2. Oil: To soften feces or to soothe irritated mucous membranes.

Prescriptions usually ordered

1. The food most likely to be absorbed:
   a. Peptonized milk.
   b. Dextrose.
   c. Beef peptones.
   d. Egg, whole or just the white.
2. Oil solutions usually ordered:
   a. Olive oil, 6 ounces.
   b. Castor oil, 2 ounces, and glycerine, 2 ounces.

Temperature of solutions

1. 105° F. for both oil and nutritive enemata.

General instructions for nutritive enema

1. Utmost patience and skill should be used to secure the best possible results.
2. Patient must be free from all causes of mental excitement, and of physical discomforts and unrest.
3. Condition of the bowel must be clean and healthy.
4. Foods must be predigested.
5. Small amounts only should be given.
6. Injections should be given slowly.
7. After injection, the patient should be kept as quiet and comfortable as possible.

Necessary articles for above enemata

Same as for emollient enema.

Record

1. Hour and treatment.
2. Formula and amount.
3. Whether retained or expelled.
4. Length of time retained.

Anthelmintic, Antiseptic, Astringent, and Saline Enemata

Aim
1. Anthelmintic: To destroy worms.
2. Antiseptic: To destroy bacteria.
3. Astringent: To contract the tissues and blood vessels.
4. To provide the body with fluid.

Prescriptions usually ordered
1. Anthelmintic:
    a. Infusion of quassia, 6 ounces.
    b. Tannic acid, 30 grains, and hot water, 1 pint.
2. Antiseptic:
    a. Silver nitrate.
    b. Alum.
    c. Tannic acid.

General instructions
1. The patient should be encouraged to retain the anthelmintic solution for from 15 to 30 minutes.

Temperature of solution
1. Anthelmintic: 105° F.; astringent: 120° F.; saline: 105° F.

Necessary articles
1. Anthelmintic: Same as for carminative enema.
2. Antiseptic: Same as for carminative enema.
3. Astringent: Same as for carminative enema.
4. Saline: Same as for emollient enema.

Procedure
1. Anthelmintic: Same as for carminative enema.
2. Antiseptic: Same as for carminative enema.
3. Astringent: Same as for carminative enema.
4. Saline: a. Same as for emollient enema.
    b. In the form of enteroclysis and proctoclysis.

Record
1. Hour and treatment.
2. Formula and amount.
3. Whether retained or expelled; results.

Enteroclysis, or Colon Irrigation

Aim
1. To thoroughly cleanse the large intestines.
2. To stimulate peristalsis and relieve flatulence.
3. To supply heat as a stimulant in shock or collapse.
4. To supply fluid to the body.

Solutions commonly used
1. Physiological salt solution.
2. Plain water.
3. Soda bicarbonate 1 to 5 per cent.
4. Starch solution.
5. Flaxseed solution.

Temperature of solution
1. For absorption: Between 100° and 110° F.
2. For inflammation: Between 115° and 120° F.
3. For cleansing: 100°—105° F.

Amount of solution
1. This depends upon the duration of the treatment.

Duration of treatment
1. From fifteen minutes to several hours.

Necessary articles
Same as for cleansing enema with the exception of the solution which may be stated in order.

Procedure
1. Prepare articles and patient the same as for cleansing enema.
2. Give the same as cleansing enema except use a rectal tube and introduce 2 to 3 inches.
3. Unless the solution is to be absorbed, encourage the patient to retain it for 15 to 20 minutes.
4. After solution has been expelled, repeat, giving the same amount.
5. Continue until the solution returns clear.
6. Two or three injections are usually necessary.
7. When treatment is finished, care for the patient in the usual way.

Care of articles
1. Same as in cleansing enema.

Record
1. Hour and treatment.
2. Amount and kind of solutions used.
3. Character of return flow.

Colon Irrigation

Minneapolis General Hospital

Aim
1. After operations:
   a. To cleanse the large intestine of excess mucus, feces, and toxic, putrefying matter.
   b. To stimulate peristalsis and relieve flatulence.

c. To supply heat as a stimulant in cases of shock or collapse.
d. To supply fluid.
2. To relieve constipation.
3. In obstruction.
4. In dysentery, to cleanse from mucus and pus and to dilute toxins.
5. To supply local remedies in inflammatory diseases of the lining of the intestines.
6. To relieve inflammation of the kidneys and pelvic viscera.
7. To relax the muscles and relieve pain in colic, hepatic, biliary, or renal.
8. To dilute and help eliminate the poisons in toxemia and uremic poisoning.
9. In poisoning from bichloride of mercury.

Necessary articles

Standard.
Irrigating can, 3 feet rubber tubing, clamp, connecting tip with small rectal tube attached for inflow.
Medium sized rectal tube for outflow. This should reach into bed pan for return flow one foot below level of mattress. If not long enough a connecting tip and rubber tubing of sufficient length should be attached.
Note: The inlet tube should be inserted about six inches while the outlet tube is inserted about three or three and one-half inches. Mark each tube with a narrow strip of adhesive to indicate when the tube has been inserted the desired distance.
Emesis basin.
Lubricant.
Toilet paper.
Rubber protector and cover large enough to be placed under patient and protect side of the bed.
Bed pan and cover.
Solution as ordered—Temperature 116°-120°.
Blanket (it is essential to keep the patient warm).

Procedure

1. Place articles on a tray.
2. Cover bed pan. Put tray on top of pan and carry to bedside together.
3. Screen patient.
4. Draw patient well to the side of the bed in the left Sim's position.
Note: If necessary, treatment may be given with the patient lying on his back with hips elevated. Right Sim's position and knee-chest position are sometimes ordered for this treatment.

5. Put blanket over patient and turn bedclothes down below waist line.
6. Protect bed with rubber sheet and cover.
7. Put bed pan on chair in position for return flow.
8. Hang can filled with solution on standard.
9. Allow solution to run through tubing to expel air and to warm tubing.
10. Place small tube in opening in side of large tube and lubricate. Insert as one tube. Adjust tubes so each is inserted the desired distance as indicated by markers on tube. Outflow tube should be about one foot below the level of the patient in order to avoid too great suction.
11. Allow solution to run slowly and with an even flow. If patient complains of pain shut off flow for a few seconds. If given properly there should be no pain. If pain is continuous stop treatment. Stop treatment if patient shows signs of exhaustion.
12. When desired effect has been attained, remove tubes gently.
13. Cleanse patient and remove rubber protector and cover. If parts are irritated, apply a soothing ointment.
14. Straighten bedclothes and leave patient comfortable.
15. Remove all articles from bedside.

Care of articles used

1. Wash and dry irrigating can and tubing.
2. Wash rectal tubes first in cold water; then in warm water and soap.
3. Boil rectal tubes for three minutes.

Record

1. Amount and kind of solution used.
2. Character of return flow.
3. Whether or not the treatment caused pain.

LESSON XXVI
PROCTOCLYSIS

Aim

1. To supply the body with fluid.

Necessary articles

Standard.
Irrigating can and double tubing.
Rectal tube or catheter, size Fr. 18, 10, Am. 12.
Vaseline and paper square for applying.
Narrow adhesive strip for securing tube if patient is restless.
Hot water bags (2) or some special apparatus as the Meineke heater.
Bed-pan cover.
Rubber protector.
Kidney basin.

Solutions usually ordered

1. Tap water.
2. Physiological salt solution.
3. Glucose solution 5 per cent, and sodium bicarbonate solution 2-5 per cent.

Procedure

1. Prepare solution ordered at 105° F.
2. Carry the articles to the bedside and screen the patient.
3. Hang can on the standard about 2 feet above the bed.
4. Place the patient in a comfortable position.
5. Place bed-pan cover and rubber protector under patient.
6. Attach the catheter, and lubricate about 6 inches of it.
7. Open the stopcock and fill the tube with the warm solution.
8. Close the stopcock and following directions in previous demonstration, introduce the tube 4 to 6 inches.
9. If the patient is restless, secure the tube by winding a narrow strip of adhesive 10 inches long once around catheter and fasten the ends to either hip.
10. Establish drip, 40 to 60 drops a minute.
11. It is always advisable to start the solution at 60 drops per minute and watch the tube to see whether the solution is being absorbed. Regulate accordingly.
12. Fill the hot water bags at 135° F.
13. Place on the side of the bed with the tube between (see diagram).
14. Draw a bath towel or small woolen blanket around both and pin. This makes the tube secure and the patient is assured against being burned. If the bags are well covered by the

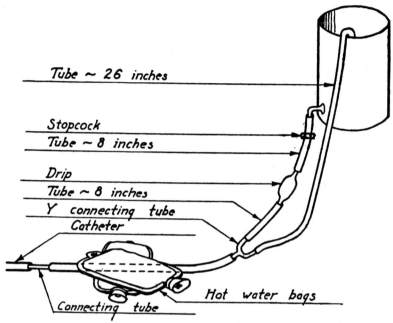

bedclothing they will retain the heat for hours and the solution in the tube will be kept at body temperature for that time.

15. The treatment may be continuous or it may be stopped every 2 or 3 hours. A favorite method is to give for 2 or 3 hours.
16. When discontinuing for a short time the flow may be stopped by the stopcock. If for 2 hours or longer, withdraw the tube, disconnect, and clean.
17. To record, record on chart when started and when discontinued. Record amounts on slip on chart. The total for the 24 hours is recorded by the night nurse.

Sample of Slip on Chart

Time	Amount added	Expelled (estimated)	Amount in can	Amount taken
4 P. M.	1000 cc.			
8 P. M.	1000 cc.	200 cc.		800 cc.
4 A. M.	500 cc.			1000 cc.
6 A. M.			200 cc.	300 cc.
Total	2500 cc.	200 cc.	200 cc.	2100 cc.

Care of articles

1. Clean thoroughly, boil catheter, drain and dry, replace in box in good condition. Leave can clean and dry.

LESSON XXVII
LOCAL APPLICATIONS FOR THE RELIEF OF INFLAMMATION AND CONGESTION
Fomentations

Aim
1. To relieve pain and congestion in the adjoining parts.
2. To relieve pain and congestion in internal organs.
3. To relieve tympanites.
4. To reduce a swelling.
5. To stimulate the absorption of exudates.

General instructions
1. Avoid chilling the part before, during, or after the treatment.
2. Apply one fomentation as the other is removed.
3. Do not use turpentine in fomentations applied for the relief of pain or congestion of the kidneys.
4. Use great care to prevent the skin being burned.

Necessary articles
Bath blanket.
Stupe tray with:
  Basin.
  Stupe wringer and sticks.
  Two pieces of flannel (twice the size of the abdomen).
  Safety pins.
  Piece of oiled muslin or waxed paper (to cover the wet flannel).
  Olive oil (2 drams).
  Applicators with cotton.
  Cotton balls (2).
  Castile or ivory soap.
  Small dressing bowl.
  Hot water bottle and cover.
  Binder, triangular bandage, bandage, or bath towel, depending on area to be treated.
  Towel.

Preparation
1. Place one flannel in stupe wringer and place in basin.
2. Fill basin with water, being sure that stupe wringer is well covered.
3. Place basin in sterilizer or over a flame and heat until the material has become thoroughly hot and steaming.
4. Prepare the hot water bottle for use and place it between the folds of a towel.
5. Remove basin and wring flannel dry with stupe wringer.
6. Pour out water and place stupe wringer with flannel in basin.

7. Cover with oiled muslin or waxed paper and dry flannel.
8. Arrange all articles on the tray and carry to the bedside.

Procedure

1. Applied to abdomen:
   a. Screen the patient.
   b. Fold the gown back and cover the abdomen with the warmed towel.
   c. Turn the bath blanket back over the chest and place the oiled muslin or waxed paper over the edge of the upper bedclothes.
   d. Pass the binder under the patient.
   e. Apply olive oil to the area with the cotton applicators.
   f. Remove wet flannel from wringer, shake once, and apply quickly to area. Be sure that flannel is wrung dry.
   g. Cover with oiled muslin or waxed paper and then with dry flannel.
   h. Arrange binder or whatever is used to hold fomentation in place.
   i. Place hot water bag.
   j. Arrange bedclothes.
   k. Second fomentation prepared in the same way, before the first one is removed.
   l. Renew in fifteen minutes or as often as ordered.
   m. Renew olive oil before every third application.
   n. When fomentations are discontinued sponge area with cotton, soap, and warm water. Pat dry and apply dry flannel.
   o. Remove tray. Clear and put articles in proper places.
2. Turpentine stupes or fomentations:
   Apply them in the same manner as simple hot water fomentations or stupes, plus the use of turpentine, which increases the counterirritant effect.
   Mix the turpentine and oil in a medicine glass (1 dram of turpentine to 7 drams of olive oil), heat by letting stand in a basin of hot water. Apply in the same way as the olive oil. Apply this mixture before every third application according to the reddening of the skin.
3. Applied for purely local effect such as:
   a. Infected finger.
   b. Boil, etc.
   c. The application should not be larger than necessary.
   d. Hold in place with bath towel, bandage, or triangular bandage.
4. Applied to breast:
   a. Cut a hole in center of stupe cloths to prevent nipple being covered.
   b. Hold in place with breast binder.

Cold Compresses for the Head

Aim
1. To relieve congestion or pain in the head.
2. To reduce temperature.

General instructions
1. Avoid allowing the water to drop from the compresses.
2. Do not allow the patient to become chilled.

Necessary articles
Tray with:
A medium sized basin fixed the same as for eye compresses.
Piece of ice about size of basin, flat on top.
Face towel.
Rubber protector.
2 compresses 8" or 9" x 4", made of four thicknesses of loosely
woven cotton material. Fold with raw edges turned in.

Preparation
1. Place table at head of bed to the right of the patient.
2. Cover basin with piece of gauze.
3. Make gauze taut by tying corners under the edge of the basin.
4. Place ice on gauze.
5. Wet the 2 compresses and wring them out as dry as possible
and place them on ice.
6. Carry the tray to the bedside.

Procedure
1. Cover rubber protector with the towel and place under the
patient's head.
2. Be sure that the patient's hair is brushed well away from the
forehead.
3. Place a compress from the ice across the forehead close to
the eyes but not over them.
4. Change compresses every 5 minutes.
5. Continue for 30 minutes or as directed.

Record
1. Hour and treatment.
2. Duration of treatment.
3. Result of treatment

LESSON XXVIII
LOCAL APPLICATIONS FOR THE RELIEF OF INFLAM-
MATION AND CONGESTION, Continued
Flaxseed Poultices

Aim

1. To relieve pain and congestion in pneumonia.
2. To stimulate the absorption of inflammatory products in pneumonia.
3. To hasten suppuration in infections.

General instructions

1. Have the poultice as light as possible.
2. Have the poultice as hot as can be borne without burning the patient.
3. Avoid exposure of the part during or after the treatment.
4. Never permit the poultice to remain on longer than an hour.
5. Be sure that the poultice is large enough to completely cover the area.

Necessary articles

Boiling water (3 cups).
Flaxseed (2 cups). Amount depends on size of poultice.
Gauze, thin muslin, or any soft material on which to spread poultice, double the size of finished poultice.
Oiled muslin.
Large board or heavy paper.
Face towel.
Saucepan and large spoon or spatula for preparation.
Flannel.
Stove or grill.
Sodium bicarbonate.
Tray with:
    Binder, triangular bandage, bandage, or bath towel, depending on the area to be treated.
    Safety pins.
    Olive oil (2 drams) warmed.
    Applicators with cotton.
    Small dressing bowl.
    Receptacle for waste.
    Castile or ivory soap.
    Cotton balls.

Preparation

1. Put the water on to boil.
2. Spread a towel on the board or heavy paper.

3. Place flannel, oiled muslin, and thin muslin (fold as for mustard plaster) in center of towel.
4. When the water is boiling add the flaxseed to it, stirring the mixture with a spoon or spatula.
5. Make the mixture just thick enough to drop from spoon.
6. When it is the right consistency, remove from the fire and add 1 teaspoonful of sodium bicarbonate. Beat until light.
7. Spread it evenly on the muslin foundation about ¼ to ½ inch thick.
8. Fold poultice to meet center and fold one end into the other.
9. Roll together, towel, flannel, oiled muslin, and poultice.
10. Wash articles used.
11. Carry with other articles on a tray to the bedside.

Procedure
1. Screen the patient.
2. Slip binder under patient beneath the part to be poulticed.
3. Arrange bedclothing and gown so that they will be out of the way.
4. Using cotton applicators, paint area with olive oil.
5. Cover area with the towel that is around the poultice.
6. Test the temperature of the poultice on back of hand and slip it under towel.
7. Put poultice on slowly so as to accustom patient to the heat.
8. Cover with flannel and oiled muslin.
9. Remove the towel and pin the binder.
10. Change every hour or as ordered.

Method of changing
1. Make fresh poultice exactly the same as the first.
2. Roll in towel and carry to the bedside.
3. Unfasten binder and slip the used poultice from underneath the oiled muslin.
4. Apply fresh poultice the same as the first.

To remove when discontinued
1. Sponge area with cotton, soap, and warm water.
2. Pat dry with cotton.

Record
1. Time and treatment.
2. Method of application.
3. Results and patient's reaction to the treatment.

Mustard Plasters

Aim
1. To relieve cerebral congestion, headache, and neuralgia, or congestion in pleurisy and pneumonia.

2. To relieve nausea and pain in the stomach.
3. To relieve abdominal pain due to flatulence and congestion.

Necessary articles

Mustard.
Flour.
Dish and spoon.
Tepid water.
Thin muslin cloth a little more than twice the size ordered.
Face towel.
Hot water bottle, warm plate, or warm basin.
Tray with:
    3 cotton balls.
    Small basin.
    Oiled muslin the size of the plaster.
    Castile or ivory soap.
    Olive oil (2 drams) warmed.
    Applicators with cotton.

Preparation

1. Fold face towel, place oiled muslin on towel.
2. Fold old muslin thus: two opposite edges creased to center and ends folded in.
3. Place folded muslin on board or newspaper.
4. Take mustard and flour
   For adult: 1 part mustard to 6 parts flour.
   For child: 1 part mustard to 12 parts flour.
5. Mix with tepid water.
6. Mix well to insure that there are no lumps of mustard.
7. Make a paste thick enough to spread without running.
8. Spread paste about ½ inch thick on muslin.
9. Insert the third edge into the sides already folded, thus making all even. If desired, the edges may be basted with long stitches.
10. Place the plaster on a hot water bottle, a warm plate, or warm basin, covered with the oiled muslin and towel.
11. Carry with other articles to the bedside on a small tray.

Procedure

1. Screen the patient.
2. Prepare patient the same as for flaxseed poultice.
3. Apply plaster to the skin and cover with oiled muslin and towel.
4. Use binder to hold in place if necessary.
5. Leave 15 or 20 minutes or until the skin is well reddened.
6. Watch the skin closely after five minutes have elapsed, for a burn from a mustard application is always the result of carelessness.

To remove

1. When the plaster is removed, sponge area with cotton, soap,

and warm water to remove particles of mustard. Pat dry with cotton. If skin is too irritated, apply vaseline or olive oil and cover with muslin.

Record

1. Time and treatment.
2. Method of application.
3. Results and patient's reaction to treatment.

Other Applications

For the application of the following in the treatment of inflammation and congestion, note the following references:

Chemical rubefacients .... Harmer, *Principles and Practice of Nursing*, pp. 329-334.

Mechanical rubefacients .... Harmer, *Principles and Practice of Nursing*, pp. 334-338 and 345-346; Kelley, *Textbook of Nursing Technique*, pp. 168-170.

Physical rubefacients;
the thermo-cautery .... Harmer, *Principles and Practice of Nursing*, pp. 327-328; Kelley, *Textbook of Nursing Technique*, pp. 171-172.

Local application of
dry heat; a hot water bag ...... Harmer, *Principles and Practice of Nursing*, pp. 199-203.

Local applications of cold....... Harmer, *Principles and Practice of Nursing*, pp. 216-220.

Vesicants, epispastics, or
blisters .... Harmer, *Principles and Practice of Nursing*, pp. 338-341.

Escharotics or caustics .... Harmer, *Principles and Practice of Nursing*, pp. 341-342.

Depletion, blood-letting, or decreasing the volume of blood,
leeching. .... Harmer, *Principles and Practice of Nursing*, pp. 342-345; Kelley, *Textbook of Nursing Technique*, pp. 340-341.

LESSON XXIX

THE HOT FOOT BATH

Aim

1. To reduce inflammation or congestion in remote or local parts.
2. For cleansing purposes.

Necessary articles

Foot tub ½ full of water, 110°-115° F. or temperature ordered.
Bath blanket.
2 bath towels.
Hot water bottle and cover.
Rubber sheet.
Pitcher of hot water.
Bath thermometer.

Procedure when patient is in bed

1. Assemble articles at the bedside.
2. Screen the patient.
3. Loosen the upper bedclothes at the foot of the bed.
4. Flex the patient's knees.
5. Fold back upper covers approximately two feet from the lower edge of the mattress being sure that the feet are kept covered.
6. Place bath blanket over rubber sheet.
7. Place upper edge of bath towel even with center of bath blanket.
8. Fold blanket and rubber sheet crosswise.
9. Place this across the foot of the bed.
10. Fanfold upper half of blanket and rubber sheet.
11. Put your arm nearest the head of the bed under the knees, and draw rubber sheet, bath blanket, and bath towel up under patient's thighs.
12. Fold back upper bedclothes to knees, pulling up bath blanket at the same time.
13. Place tub lengthwise near the feet.
14. Fold back corner of blanket.
15. Put your arm nearest the head of the bed under patient's legs and your hand under his heels.
16. Put your other arm across the tub, grasp it on the far side, and move it forward into position, while at the same time you raise the feet and legs from the bed. This is done under the top layer of the blanket; the arm being kept across the tub to prevent the blanket getting into the water.
17. Place the patient's feet in the tub slowly, heels first.
18. Place the bath towel folded over rim of tub between patient's legs and the tub.
19. Bring rubber sheet up over blanket and knees.

20. Place the hot water bottle under the blanket.
21. Take hold of the upper edge of the blanket and hold it in position, while with your other hand draw down the covers.
22. The feet are kept in the water from fifteen to twenty minutes.
23. If it is necessary to raise the temperature of the water, pour in hot water from the pitcher slowly, keeping your hand between the patient's legs and the stream. This can be done without uncovering the tub except at the point where you are pouring in the water.
24. To remove the tub, turn covers back above knees.
25. Put your arm under the legs as when putting the feet in the tub.
26. Pull the tub toward you and place the feet on the bath towel.
27. Remove the tub.
28. Dry the feet with bath towel under the feet.
29. Remove the blanket and rubber sheet and pull down upper covers.
30. Place hot water bottle at the feet.
31. Tuck covers under mattress as usual.

Record
1. Hour and treatment.
2. Duration of treatment.
3. Any unusual symptoms.

Care of articles
1. See that all articles used in the treatment are cared for and returned to the proper place.
   Note: If mustard is ordered, it should be mixed with water and the paste added to the tub of water, or it may be put in a small gauze bag and placed in the tub of water. Use about two tablespoonfuls of mustard to a gallon of water.

ADVANCED PRACTICAL NURSING

LESSON I
THE ADMINISTRATION OF MEDICINES

Responsibilities of the nurse

1. Administration of medicines is one of the most responsible duties assigned to student nurses.
2. The nurse should see that medication is received by patient accurately, promptly, and in such a way as to give best results.
3. She should know:
   a. The nature of the drug.
   b. To what its action (local and systemic) is due.
   c. Maximum and minimum dosage.
   d. Factors that modify dosage and its effect:
      (1) Age.
      (2) Sex.
      (3) Previous habits or toleration.
      (4) Idiosyncrasy.
      (5) Temperament and occupation.
      (6) Condition of patient.
      (7) Nature and form of medication.
      (8) Object of medication.
      (9) Time of administration.
      (10) Channel of administration.
   e. Disease from which patient is suffering.
   f. The effect desired.
   g. Why the drug is being given.
   h. Symptoms which indicate the desired and possible undesired results.
   i. Symptoms of over dosage.
   j. Idiosyncrasy.
   k. Cumulative poisoning.
   l. "Physiologic limit."
   m. Treatment for poisoning.
   n. Drug habit:
      (1) Necessity for decreasing the use of drugs gradually.
      (2) Means of restricting use of drugs.
   o. Never be mechanical in the administration of drugs.
   p. Always ask the physician what the prescription contains.

The medicine cupboard

1. Keep medicine case locked. Do not leave key in lock. Carry the key.
2. Arrange drugs in medicine case with bottles of same size together and with all the more powerful drugs apart from others and in bottles with a rough exterior or other distinguishing feature and marked poison.
3. Keep oils in a cool place.

4. Keep vaccines in ice box.
5. Never have medicine in unmarked bottles. Never change the label on a bottle—have the druggist do it. Keep labels clean.
6. Never order a large amount of drugs because some deteriorate.
7. Keep all bottles corked tightly. Some may contain volatile substances and will become either stronger or weaker if left uncorked.
8. Keep shelves and bottles clean.
9. The rim of the bottle should always be cleaned after pouring.
10. Leave the medicine case ready for the next giving of medicine.
11. Leave sink clean.
12. Any change in color, odor, or consistency of medicines should be reported.
13. Report shortage of drugs to head nurse.
14. Return special prescription to drug room when medicine is discontinued.

The medicine tray

1. Articles necessary:
   Tray with:
      Medicine glasses.
      Minim glass.
      Stirring rod.
      Medicine dropper.
      Pitcher.
2. Instructions:
   a. Return glasses to tray after the giving of medicines. Do not leave on patient's tray or in room.
   b. Leave tray clean and filled with glasses, etc., for next hour.
   c. Leave sink clean and leave clean towels on rack.
   d. Always wipe off edge of bottle before replacing on shelf after pouring medicine.

Duties of the Medicine Nurse

Minneapolis General Hospital

General instructions

1. Be accurate in all things. These are responsible duties and may mean the life of the patient if errors are made.
2. Systematize and plan your work. Only one nurse is to do these duties, therefore there is more need of system.

Duties

1. The medicine and temperature nurse goes on duty at 6:40 A. M. This enables her to take the A. M. temperatures before breakfast is served.
2. The daily requisition for drugs is made out. Take a careful invoice of all drugs each morning and order current drugs or

any new ones needed. In ordering, state amount and name of drug plainly. Take drug order to head nurse to be signed. put empty containers in drug basket, also bottles of drugs no longer needed in medicine closet. Aim to order everything needed for the day. If necessary to send in a requisition during the day, it must be signed at the School of Nursing office.

3. Orders for morphine from drug room must be accompanied by the Morphine Record Sheet. Ten tablets of the same strength are issued at one time. As morphine is given in the ward, it must be recorded immediately on record sheet. Day nurse records in black ink. Night nurse in red ink. The morphine tablets on hand and the morphine given must balance with the amount issued.

4. After giving medicines, take trays with glasses to the kitchen to have the maid wash them.

5. Abnormal pulses should be charted and reported to the head nurse.

6. Any symptoms observed that may be the result of medicines given should be charted by medicine and temperature nurse.

7. Doctor's order book:
   a. All orders for patients are written by the doctor in the order book.
   b. These are copied on patient's chart on order sheet by medicine and temperature nurse.
   c. The day nurse on medicine and temperatures copies all orders in black ink and all must be copied before going off duty. After copying on chart a "C" is marked through order.
   d. At 7 P. M. a line is drawn across order book with hour and date in black ink.
   e. The night nurse copies all orders written at night in red ink and at 7 A. M. a red line is drawn across the order book with hour and date.

8. Charting:
   a. Chart medicines only when given, for example, Tr. dig. m XV t. i. d. at 8-12-5 (the hours 8-12-5 are to be filled in as given).
   b. Medications given hypodermically should be charted as follows: Morph. gr. ⅛ (H).

9. Before going off duty:
   a. The medicine closet must be in perfect order, hypodermic tray and medicine trays equipped.
   b. All medicines that might be needed for night must be in stock.
   c. All charting must be done.
   d. All orders must be copied.

Rules for the Giving of Medicines

(Medicine case must be kept locked)

General instructions

1. Never speak to anyone or allow anyone to speak to you while giving medicine.
2. Always give *exactly* what is ordered, *on time.*
3. Give *minims* when *minims* are ordered. *Drops* when *drops* are ordered.
4. Read the label on the bottle *three times*:
   a. Before taking from the shelf.
   b. Before pouring from the bottle.
   c. After pouring from the bottle.
5. Always shake bottle before pouring out medicine.
6. While pouring medicine, hold bottle with label on upper side to avoid defacing it. Before replacing the bottle, wipe rim with gauze kept for that purpose.
7. While pouring, hold glass with mark of the quantity you require on the level with your eye.
8. Always recork bottles immediately after use.
9. Give acids and medicines containing iron through a glass tube.
10. *Never* allow one patient to carry medicine to another.
11. *Never* record a dose as given until patient has actually taken it.
12. Never use medicine when you are in doubt as to the nature of its contents, or medicine from an unmarked bottle.
13. Never mix or give at the same time, medicines in which there is a chemical change when put together, unless with the knowledge and direction of the physician.
14. A change in color, odor, or consistency of any substance should be reported and a fresh supply obtained.
15. The nurse in charge of the medicine cabinet is responsible for the examination of medicines daily. She should order drugs in such quantity as will insure the drugs being fresh.
16. Any nurse giving medicine is entirely responsible for the taking of it by the patient.
17. She is to see that water is provided bed patients to take with medicine.
18. She is to stand by any patient who has to be wakened and see that medicine is taken.
19. She must not leave bedside of ill patients until medicine is taken.
20. When patients refuse to take medicine it must be reported and recorded on chart.
21. Remember there is an element of danger in every drop of medicine.
22. Read your orders carefully and be sure that you understand them.
23. Never give a drug in the dark or in the dim light.

24. Never give a medicine about which you have a shadow of doubt; find out about it.
25. When giving liquid medicines to an unconscious patient, drop it far back on the tongue, using a dessert spoon.
26. Never place a pill or powder on the tongue of a delirious or unconscious patient. Dissolve in water and give.
27. No medicine is to be kept in the medicine cupboard in an unlabeled medicine glass.
28. Never give medicine to a patient when the medicine has been prepared by another nurse.

Rules for giving medicines with the card system

1. Cards are marked with patient's name, medication, dose, time, date, and nurse's initials.
2. Cards must be clean and legible.
3. Medication to be given by "hypo" must be so stated on the card. Sample of card:

> Mr. John Brown
> Tr. digitalis m. V—t.i.d.
> 8/12/5
> 2-4-28   H.M.T.

4. Arrange cards according to colors in pockets.
5. Cards are made out by medicine nurse or by nurse instructed to do so according to routine of the hospital from doctor's order book and left on head nurse's desk. She checks the order and places card in medicine card box. At night the night supervisor does this. When the medications are to be given out, the nurse places the cards in a row, and as the medication is prepared, attaches the card to the glass and does not remove it until the medicine is given to the patient. After medication is discontinued, card is bent by medicine nurse and left on head nurse's desk. The head nurse checks the order and destroys the card.
6. Medicine list:

> Q.3.h. . . . . .pink.
> Q.4.h. . . . . .red.
> A.c. t.i.d. . . . . .blue.
> P.c. t.i.d. . . . . .yellow.
> Irregular orders . . . .green.
> Treatment . . . . .white.
> Q.h. . . . . . . .one corner off.
> Q.2.h. . . . . .one corner off.
> Q.6.h. . . . . .one corner off.
> B.i.d. . . . . . .one corner off.

Hours of administration

4.i.d.—8 A. M., 12 N., 4 P. M., and 8 P.M.
Q. 2 h.—6, 8, 10, 12, etc.

Q. 3 h.—9, 12, 3, 6, etc.
Q. 4 h.—8, 12, 4, etc.
Q. 6 h.—6, 12, etc.
B.i.d.—8 A. M., 4 P. M.
T.i.d.—8, 12-5.
A.c.—½ hour before meals.
P.c.—½ hour after meals.
O.d. daily—10 A. M.
O.m. each morning—6 A. M.
O.n. each night—8 P. M.

Channels of administration
1. How given:
   a. Mouth.
   b. Subcutaneously.
   c. Per rectum.
   d. Inunction.
   e. Inhalation.
   f. Intravenously, e. g., salvarsan.
   g. Hypodermoclysis, e. g., normal saline.
   h. Intramuscular injection, e. g., mercury salicylate.
2. Order of absorption:
   a. Subcutaneously.
   b. Inhalation—due to the number of blood vessels in the lungs.
   c. By mouth.
   d. Per rectum.
   e. Inunction.

Administration by Mouth

General instructions
1. Make the dose as palatable as possible.
2. Use either very hot or very cold water.

Pills and capsules
1. Place well back on tongue and follow with sufficient amount of water to enable patient to swallow medicine comfortably.

Oils
1. Give in wines, fruit juices, coffee, etc.

Iron and acids
1. Always give with glass tube. The action of iron and acids destroys enamel on teeth.

Cough syrups
1. Do not add water, it destroys action of drug, which is not soothing to mucous membrane if diluted.

Powders
1. Give in syrup, glycerine, jam, honey, or place on back of tongue.

Salines
1. Do not dilute unless they are given for the purpose of getting fluid into the body and for stimulation.

Calomel
1. Do not give milk or eggs just before or after calomel as they combine to form albuminate of mercury.
2. Do not give salt, or food containing it, near calomel. It combines to form a poisonous compound.

Croton oil
8. May be given on sugar or in prepared olive oil.

Administration of Suppositories

Aim
1. To introduce drugs into the rectum for a direct local effect.

Kinds of suppositories
1. Concentrated food.
2. Soap.
3. Glycerine.
4. Plain or medicated cocoa butter.

Necessary articles
Suppository.
Gauze squares.
Tube of vaseline.
Finger cot or rectal tube.

Procedure
1. Place the suppository on a piece of gauze and lubricate it.
2. Carry articles to the bedside.
3. Screen the patient.
4. Turn the patient on his left side if possible, otherwise he may be in the dorsal recumbent position.
5. Nurse is to cover index finger with rubber cot. Lubricate finger with vaseline.
6. Pass suppository into the rectum beyond the internal sphincter muscle. The suppository can be pushed in with a rectal tube instead of using finger with finger cot.
7. Apply pressure over the anus for a few moments until the patient has no desire to expel the suppository.

Chart
1. Hour.
2. Kind of suppository.
3. Length of time retained, if the patient expels it.
4. Patient's reaction.

Inunctions

Aim

1. To administer a drug through the skin.

Medications most commonly applied

1. Cod-liver oil.
2. Olive oil.
3. Cocoa butter.
4. Mercurial ointment.

Necessary articles for applying cod-liver oil, olive oil, or cocoa butter

Wash basin containing warm water.
Soap.
Bath towel.
Medication.

Areas to which application may be made

Chest, abdomen, back, limbs, whole body.

Procedure

1. Screen the patient.
2. Cleanse the skin with hot water and soap and dry.
3. Warm the oil.
4. Rub oil in with the palm of the hand until absorbed.
5. Use a circular movement.

Application of mercurial ointment

1. In addition to the above necessary articles use:
   a. Rubber glove.
   b. Piece of old muslin to wipe ointment from glove.
   c. Newspaper.
2. Procedure
   a. Screen the patient.
   b. Select a portion of the body and cleanse. Consult head nurse in regard to the portions of the body that are used for the "course" of treatments.
   c. Protect the bed with newspaper.
   d. Put on rubber glove and apply ointment to exposed area. Rub it into the skin thoroughly by using a rotary motion.
   e. Apply the ointment in this way for five days, using a different surface each day.
   f. Do not give the treatment on the sixth day.
   g. Give the patient a bath on the seventh day and then continue the treatment as before.

Record

1. Hour.
2. Medication.
3. Site of application.

Inhalations

Aim
1. To relieve spasmodic breathing.
2. To disinfect bronchial secretions.
3. To stimulate expectoration.
4. To afford comfort to the patient.

General instructions
1. If the patient is to be kept quiet, as in pneumonia, and the towel and pitcher method is used, the nurse must hold the pitcher.
2. If the patient is up and around, all steam inhalations should be given at bed time. If the treatment is ordered during the day, the patient should not be permitted to go out for at least an hour afterward.
3. Avoid drafts.
4. In whatever method used, great care must be taken that the patient is not burned.
5. If a canopy is used, arrange it so that there will be ample ventilation and so that it will present a neat appearance.

Methods of giving inhalations
1. Pitcher and towel method.
2. Teakettle and cone with electric plate.
3. Inhaler.
4. Croup tent (taught in pediatric nursing).

Medications and treatments given by inhalation
1. Tr. benzoin dr. 1 to 1 pt. boiling water.
2. Anesthetics:
   a. Ether.
   b. Oxygen gas.
   c. Chloroform.
3. Aromatic spirits of ammonia:
   a. Saturate a piece of gauze and hold to patient's nose.
   b. Usually given in syncope.
4. Amyl nitrite pearls:
   a. Never given without a doctor's order. Given as a stimulant.
   b. Crush the pearl in a piece of gauze and allow patient to inhale vapor.
   c. Care must be taken not to hold too close to the nose, as it may cause epistaxis.
5. Stramonium leaves:
   a. Given as dry inhalation.
   b. The drug is placed on a heated plate and fumes inhaled through a cone.
6. Steam.

Pitcher and towel method

1. Necessary articles:
   Bath blanket.
   Medication.
   Boiling water.
   Bath towel.
   Face towel.
   Large hand basin.
2. Preparation:
   a. Pour prescribed drug into pitcher of boiling water (always use an old pitcher).
   b. Fold a bath towel in thirds crosswise and wrap around pitcher so as to prevent patient from being burned and to form funnel through which vapor can be inhaled.
3. Procedure:
   a. Prepare the patient. If he is convalescing he may sit up and take the treatment himself, or three pillows may be placed under his head.
   b. Fasten a bath blanket around patient's shoulders.
   c. Assist patient to one side of bed.
   d. Place the patient on his side with his head near the edge of the pillows.
   e. Place the pitcher of hot solution in a deep basin on the bed at the edge of the pillows.
   f. Make a canopy of the face towel.
   g. Instruct the patient to inhale through his mouth and exhale through his nose for five or six breaths and then rest a while.

Teakettle and cone

1. Necessary articles:
   Electric plate.
   Teakettle with cone or spout.
   Tent or canopy prepared according to Kelley's *Nursing Technique*, page 201.
2. Preparation:
   a. Prepare canopy.
   b. If teakettle spout has not a regular cone of metal, make one of stiff paper.
   c. Fill teakettle with water and put in medication if one is ordered.
3. Procedure:
   a. Bring articles to bedside.
   b. Attach electric plate.
   c. Place teakettle on the plate and adjust apparatus conveniently for patient to inhale steam.
   d. Be sure that inhalation outfit is absolutely secure and safe before leaving the room.
   e. Watch patient closely.

LESSON II

THE ADMINISTRATION OF MEDICINES, Continued

Administration Subcutaneously

Aim

1. To obtain prompt action of the drug.
2. To administer a drug when the patient cannot take it by mouth.
3. To prevent irritation of the mucous membrane of the stomach or rectum.
4. To obtain a reliable action.

General instructions

1. The drug must be pure and sterile.
2. All articles must be sterile, nurse's hands must be clean, and patient's skin cleansed.
3. Dissolve drug thoroughly.
4. Give oils into fleshy parts.
5. When ready to give the injection explain to the patient what you are going to do.
6. Give on outer surfaces of the arm and forearm or on the front of the thighs.
7. Occasionally a capillary is punctured which reddens an area about the site of puncture. This disappears like a bruised spot.
8. Owing to their irritating nature, give the following deep into the muscles in the gluteal or lumbar region: digitalis, quinine, bichloride of mercury, ergot, arsenic compounds.
9. Give digitalis well diluted.
10. When giving hypodermics at frequent intervals, inject into the arms or legs, always rotating in the same order giving only once in each place.

Dangers to be avoided

1. Causing an abscess.
2. Injecting a drug into a vein.
3. Breaking the needle in the tissues.

Necessary articles

Receptacle for sterile cotton pledgets.
Bottle of alcohol.
Bottle of water.
Bottle of ether (Mpls. General Hospital tray).
Alcohol lamp.
Tablespoon in which to boil water and needle.
Small forceps.
Small rubber bulb.
Medicine glass.
Sterile drug in tablet or liquid form.
Hypodermic syringe with sharp-pointed needle.

Procedure
1. Read medicine order.
2. Fill glass ½ full of alcohol.
3. Remove wire from needle and test for leakage.
4. Replace wire. Place in spoon with point toward small part of spoon. Cover with water.
5. Fill syringe with alcohol, remove plunger and let both remain in glass of alcohol.
6. Sterilize wired needle by boiling for 1 minute.
7. Rinse syringe with sterile water.
8. Flame the forceps; pick up tablet and insert into barrel.
9. Replace piston and make just enough pressure to crush the tablet.
10. Pick up needle with forceps and attach.
11. Draw up required number of minims from spoon.
12. Dissolve tablet by shaking, then express air.
13. Enfold needle in alcohol sponge.
14. Read order again.
15. Carry prepared tray to bedside.
   Note: Replace drugs and tray and lock the cupboard before going to the patient.

Method of giving
1. The safest place for hypodermic injections is on the outer surface of arms, leg, or thigh. Give here unless otherwise ordered.
2. Cleanse surface with alcohol sponge.
3. Raise tissue or draw tight between thumb and forefinger. Quickly insert the needle, slightly withdraw, then inject fluid by pressure on piston with thumb.
4. Make pressure with sponge over point of puncture.
5. Quickly withdraw needle, knead around the spot gently with the sponge.

Drugs in liquid form
1. Prepare syringe and needle to step 7.
2. Remove cork from bottle, lower needle into solution and draw into the syringe the number of minims to be given.

Care of articles used
1. Clean needle and barrel with alcohol by filling and emptying syringe.
2. Leave syringe separated and absolutely clean.
3. Dry needle thoroughly by blowing out all moisture, using rubber bulb for this purpose. At Minneapolis General Hospital ether is used to clean the needle.
4. Dry the wire before replacing in needle.
5. Leave tray in order and ready for use.

Care of tray
1. Clean every morning or as often as necessary as follows:
   a. Wash and fill bottles.
   b. Wash and boil container for cotton balls.
   c. Fill container with sterile cotton balls.
   d. Clean and fill alcohol lamp.
   e. Be sure that tray is clean and that all articles are replaced. *Tray must have all the necessary articles on it and they must be in good condition at all times.*

Record
1. Hour and treatment.
2. Drug and amount given.
3. Patient's reaction to treatment.

LESSON III

EYE, EAR, NOSE, AND THROAT TREATMENTS

Eye Irrigations

Aim

1. Cleanliness.
2. Control of infection.

General instructions

1. In cases where there is a copious discharge and Neisserian infection, the nurse should protect herself by wearing gown, rubber gloves, and in some cases the eyes may be protected by use of eyeglasses.
2. If only one eye is to be treated, protect the other eye by use of pad or dressing. If both eyes are to be treated, a sterile point should be used for each eye and the hands of the nurse scrubbed before procedure, between the care of the eyes, and after care.
3. Always direct the stream from the inner toward the outer canthus of the eye and dry with cotton, wiping in the same direction.
4. Never use force in opening eyelids, press on eyeball, nor allow the stream of solution to flow from a height more than 8 inches above the patient.
5. Do not let the tip touch the eye.
6. Be very careful that the percentage and temperature of the solution are accurate, for the cornea is very sensitive and easily irritated.

Solutions usually ordered

1. Boracic acid 2 per cent.
2. Physiological saline solution.

Temperature of solution

1. From 90° to 95° F.

Necessary articles

Medicine dropper or irrigating tip and bulb.
Rubber protector.
Solution as ordered.
Paper bag.
Kidney basin.
Towel.
Sterile cotton balls.
Safety pin.

Procedure

1. Sterilize articles necessary and prepare the tray and carry it to the bedside.

2. Bring patient to the edge of the bed or have patient seated in a chair.
3. If in bed remove all but one pillow.
4. Have head tilted slightly back and with eye to be treated slightly lower than the other to avoid washing discharge in the latter.
5. Protect the pillow and bedding with rubber protector and towel. If an up patient, fasten protector at the back of the neck.
6. Adjust kidney basin.
7. Stand behind the patient.
8. Wash off adherent discharge from the lids with pledgets moistened with solution (never put a used pledget back into the solution).
9. Separate the lids by making traction with the thumb and first finger of the left hand upon the flesh above and below the lids, exerting all necessary pressure while doing so upon the frontal and molar bones, *never on the eyeball.*
10. Have patient look up and down alternately, by moving the eyeball, not the head.
11. If unable to open lids at first, irrigate over outside until lids can be separated.
12. Dry with pledgets of cotton.
13. Care of articles after use: Thoroughly cleanse and sterilize utensils and put away.

Record
1. Hour and treatment.
2. Amount of discharge.
3. Condition of the eyes.
   Note: In cases where there is a copious discharge, and irrigations are done frequently, an irrigating can and tip can be used if ordered, in place of medicine dropper.

Administration of Eye Drops

Aim
1. To dilate the pupil.
2. To contract the pupil.
3. To relieve inflammatory conditions of the eye.
4. To produce local anesthesia preparatory to operation.

Necessary articles
Small tray with:
   Sterile medicine dropper.
   Solution.
   Sterile cotton pledgets.
   Kidney basin.

Procedure
1. Wash your hands.
2. Stand behind the patient.

3. Draw into the medicine dropper as much solution as will be required.
4. Pull down the lower lid with the index or middle finger and have the patient look up.
5. Put drop at inner canthus. Touch drop on membrane of lid before breaking off from dropper.
6. Have patient blink eyelids slowly so as to scatter the drops.
7. Put finger over opening into the tear sac in order to prevent drops getting into the nose. This is necessary for two reasons:
   a. If the medication flows into the tear sac the eye will not be as much benefitted by it as it should be.
   b. Such drugs as atropine and cocaine are sometimes applied in solutions that are strong enough to produce poisonous symptoms in children or susceptible adults if they are absorbed.
8. Do not let the dropper touch the eye.
9. Wash hands afterward to avoid applying some of the drug to your own eyes.
10. Boil dropper.

Record
1. Hour and treatment.
2. Kind and quantity of medicine instilled.

Application of Hot Compresses to the Eye

Aim
1. To relieve pain.
2. To relieve inflammation and congestion.
3. To provide comfort for the patient.

General instructions
1. Make application with a firm, sure touch, but gently.
2. Avoid pressure on the eyeball.
3. Be sure that compresses are scrupulously clean and smooth.
4. Be sure that compresses do not extend over nose or eyebrow.
5. Any discharge from eyes should be considered contagious.

Temperature of water
1. From 120° to 130° F.

Position of patient
1. Dorsal recumbent and at side of bed.

Necessary articles
1. If compresses are changed frequently:
   a. Dressing bowl of hot solution as ordered.
   b. 6 compresses of cotton slightly larger than area to be covered.
   c. Some apparatus to keep solution hot.

    d. 2 forceps.
    e. Face towel.
    f. Paper bag.
    g. Gauze square.
2. If compresses are kept hot by electric light bulb:
    a. Dressing bowl of hot solution as ordered.
    b. Compress of cotton slightly larger than area to be covered.
    c. 2 gauze squares.
    d. Extension cord with electric light bulb covered with black stocking or black cloth.
    e. 2 forceps.
    f. Face towel.
    g. Paper bag.

Procedure for compresses to be changed frequently

1. Prepare articles on tray and carry to the bedside.
2. Assist patient to side of bed.
3. Place face towel across chest.
4. If a discharging eye, protect other eye with gauze square.
5. Place compresses in hot solution.
6. Wring compress dry with forceps.
7. Apply over closed lids.
8. Change every thirty to sixty seconds for duration of time ordered, usually ten or fifteen minutes every four hours.
9. Use new compress each time. Drop used one in paper bag.
10. Repeat solution as necessary.
11. On removal, dry lids gently.
12. Clean articles on tray and replace tray on the shelf.

Procedure if compresses are kept hot by electric bulb

1. Prepare articles on tray and carry to the bedside.
2. Attach electric light extension.
3. Assist patient to side of bed.
4. Place face towel across chest.
5. Place hot compress over eye.
6. Place wet gauze square over compress.
7. Cover with dry gauze square.
8. Place covered electric light bulb in position. Support by means of pillows, or if patient is able he may hold it.
9. Leave on for 15 or 20 minutes.
10. Remove, dry eye carefully.
11. Clean articles on tray and replace tray on the shelf.

Record

1. Hour and treatment.
2. Duration of treatment.
3. Amount of discharge.

Application of Cold Compresses to the Eye

Aim

1. To relieve inflammation and congestion.

2. To relieve pain.
3. To provide comfort for the patient.

General instructions

1. The same as for hot compresses.

Position of patient

1. The same as for hot compresses.

Necessary articles

6 cotton compresses slightly larger than area to be covered.
Dressing bowl with gauze tied over the top to form a hammock for ice, or put a bowl upside down in dressing bowl and place large square of ice on it.
Face towel.
Paper bag.

Procedure

1. Prepare tray and carry to the bedside.
2. Prepare the patient as for hot compresses.
3. Moisten several cotton compresses and place on the ice.
4. Change compresses every 2 minutes. Drop used ones into bag for that purpose.
5. Use the same precautions as for hot compresses, if there is any discharge from the eyes.

Irrigation of the Ear

Aim

1. To cleanse external ear.
2. To relieve inflammation and congestion.

General instructions

1. The flow should be gentle, steady, and continuous.
2. Air bubbles should not be forced into the canal.
3. Never put a pointed instrument into the ears.
4. Never put anything cold into the ears.
5. Avoid pressure.
6. Report pain or dizziness.

Solutions usually ordered

1. Weak soda bicarbonate.
2. Normal salt solution.

Temperature of solution

105° F. for cleansing.
110° F. to relieve pain and inflammation.

Necessary articles

Irrigating can, tubing, and point.
Face towel.
Rubber protector.

Kidney basin (large).
Sterile cotton pledgets.
Sterile solution as ordered, 500 cc.

Preparation
1. Sterile irrigating can, tubing, point, and kidney basin.
2. Assemble necessary articles on a tray and carry to the bedside.

Procedure
1. Screen the patient.
2. Patient may lie down or sit up in a chair.
3. Place towel and rubber protector over the shoulder and under the ear.
4. Place kidney basin and have patient, if possible, hold it in place.
5. Place irrigator not more than one foot above the patient.
6. Connect point to rubber tubing.
7. Irrigate external ear gently.
8. Dry the ear with sterile cotton pledgets.
9. Irrigate the auditory canal gently.   Have the canal as straight as possible by holding the ear upward and backward.
10. Dry the ear thoroughly with sterile cotton pledgets.
11. Use medication as ordered.

Record
1. Hour and treatment.
2. Amount and character of the discharge.
3. Effect on the patient.

Mouth and Throat Irrigation

Aim
1. For the relief of inflammation and congestion.
2. For cleansing purposes.
3. For comfort.

Solutions usually ordered
1. Peroxide of hydrogen 25 per cent.
2. Potassium permanganate, pale wine color.
3. Physiological salt solution.
4. Sodium bicarbonate, one dram to one quart of water.
5. Boric acid 2 per cent.
6. Iron and potassium chlorate 25 per cent.
7. Dobell's solution 50 per cent.

Quantity of solution
1. One quart.

Temperature
1. From 105° to 120° F.

Position of patient
1. Semi-recumbent, near the edge of the bed, with the head turned to one side.
2. Prone.

Necessary articles
Tray with:
Irrigating can and tubing.
Connecting point with smaller tubing 12 inches long, or catheter.
Tongue depressor.
Hand basin for return flow.
Rubber sheet.
Cotton draw sheet.
Solution as ordered 110° or as hot as patient can stand it.
Safety pin.

Preparation
1. Boil irrigating can and tubing and point and tubing.
2. For a second case only the smaller tubing need be boiled.

First procedure
1. Carry tray to the bedside.
2. Place rubber sheet under head and place patient near edge of bed, with head turned on the side.
3. Place basin where it will catch the return flow.
4. Expel the air from the tube.
5. Insert tubing in mouth with right hand.
6. Press down the back part of the tongue with the rubber, but avoid touching the back part of the throat.
7. Irrigate by moving the tip from time to time so that the solution will reach all parts of the throat.
8. Continue the treatment until satisfied with the result.
9. Cleanse face and dry.

Second procedure
1. Have patient sitting up in bed or in chair.
2. Adjust rubber sheet and draw sheet about neck.
3. Place basin in patient's lap.
4. Have patient lower head over basin as throat is irrigated. Continue as in procedure I.
5. Cleanse face and dry.

Nasal Irrigations

Aim
1. To soften and remove discharges.
2. To relieve congestion, swelling, and pain.

General instructions
1. Have the irrigating can three inches above patient to prevent washing the discharge into the Eustachian tube.

2. Instruct the patient to breathe through the mouth. Be sure that the mouth is kept wide open.
3. Do not allow the patient to blow the nose or attempt to swallow while the nose is filled with solution.
4. Never place a glass tube in the nostril.

Solutions usually ordered
1. Physiological salt solution.
2. Boric acid solution.
3. Sodium bicarbonate solution.

Temperature of solution
1. 105° to 115° F.

Position of patient
1. Sitting in a chair with the head flexed on the chest.
2. Dorsal recumbent position, with head turned to side and the nostril into which the tip is inserted uppermost.

Necessary articles
Tray with:
Irrigating can and tubing.
Connecting tip with piece of ½ inch tubing 4 inches long.
Hand basin for return flow.
Rubber sheet.
Cotton sheet.
Solution as ordered.
Safety pin.
Cotton pledgets.
Gauze handkerchief for the patient.

Procedure
1. Sterilize articles and prepare tray.
2. Cover the tray and carry it to the bedside.
3. Place the patient in position.
4. Cover rubber sheet with draw sheet and fasten around patient's neck.
5. Insert the tubing just inside the nostril.
6. Irrigate the nose gently.
7. Continue the treatment until satisfied with the results, or the prescribed amount has been given.
8. Cleanse with pledgets.
9. Have the patient blow his nose, first one one side and then on the other, a short time after treatment is completed.
10. Clean and sterilize articles and replace on the shelf.

Record
1. Hour and treatment.
2. Kind, amount, and strength of solution.
3. Character of the return flow.

Nasal Irrigation

N. P. B. A. Hospital

Definition

1. A stream of plain or medicated fluid washing the nasal cavity under a low pressure.

Aim

1. To remove a thick discharge or crust.
2. To relieve congestion, swelling, or pain.

General instructions

1. Instruct the patient to breathe through his mouth and not to swallow.
2. Do not allow the patient to forcibly blow his nose after the irrigation; he may sniff out excess solution and mucus and wipe nose quietly without blowing.
3. Should not go out in the cold for at least half an hour after the irrigation.
4. Should the patient wish to swallow, stop the flow of the solution temporarily.

Necessary articles

Irrigating can with tubing, nasal douche, nozzle, catheter, or tapering glass connection protected with a piece of rubber. Standard.

Solution (105°):
   a. Normal saline.
   b. Sodium bicarbonate ½ per cent-1 per cent.
   c. Boric acid 2 per cent.

Rubber protector and towel.

Basin for return flow.

Procedure

1. Method I:
   a. Take patient to the medical dressing room; have him sit on a stool in front of the sink with head bent forward. Irrigation can 2-4 inches above the patient's nose.
   b. Pass one liter of 105° normal saline through the nostrils alternating from one to the other every 250 cc.
   c. Put about 3 drops of 10 per cent argyrol in each nostril after irrigation.
2. Method II:
   a. If the patient is a child, wrap a bath blanket around him, hold face downward, or place on a flat surface.
   b. Protect the patient with a rubber square and towel.
   c. If an adult, he may sit on a chair with his head bent forward or he may lie down in a prone position, also protect with a rubber square and towel.

d. If sitting, he may hold the basin; if reclining, place the basin on a chair or stool in front of him.

e. Insert the nozzle and tilt the head slightly, alternating sides every 250 cc.

f. Instruct patient to breathe through his mouth.

Record

1. Hour and treatment.
2. Kind and strength of solution.
3. Character and return of solution.

Care of equipment

1. Rinse equipment with cold water and boil.

LESSON IV
STERILE SUPPLIES AND TRAYS

Aim

1. To have supplies "surgically clean," that is, to prepare and handle them in such a manner as to prevent their carrying infection.

General instructions

1. Sterilized articles should never come in contact with any unsterile articles. Should an article be contaminated, it must be resterilized before using.
2. Forceps for handling sterilized materials should be cleansed, boiled, and placed in a sterile jar containing fresh cresolis compositus solution 2 per cent. This must be done daily.
3. Never allow the hand or arm to pass across an open sterile receptacle or disinfected fluid.
4. In removing sterile articles from a cover, remove the pins carefully. Never touch the inside of the cover. The contents may be removed by forceps into a sterile basin or may be dropped upon a sterile field.
5. In setting up a sterile tray, towels may be removed from the sterile package to cover the tray by picking up carefully by uppermost corner and placing over tray.
6. In holding a sterile basin, always hold by pressing the hands on the sides, or hold by placing the hands beneath the bottom of the basin; never grasp it with fingers over the rim.
7. Sterile supply jars: lift the lid straight up from the jar and remove contents with forceps. If necessary to put lid down, place with the bottom side up, so that the inner rim will not come in contact with any unsterile thing. In replacing lid, avoid striking it against the sides of the jar.
8. Sterile pitchers: keep covered with sterile towel.
9. Pouring solutions:
   a. Remove stopper from bottles without unsterilizing bottom of cork.
   b. Clean mouth of bottle with disinfectant solution on sponge, then grasp the bottle, having the label side toward the palm, and pour the solution.
   c. In case no disinfectant is available, a small amount of solution may be poured from the mouth of the bottle to cleanse the bottle, holding over a sink or basin, never over the floor.

Preparation of Trays and Care of Articles Used
University Hospital

To sterilize articles used in the various procedures

1. Tubing, stopcocks, glasses, mixing bottles, beakers, pipettes,

stirring rods, syringes, medicine droppers, small basins, etc.: Sterilize by boiling for 5 minutes.
2. Needles: Sterilize by boiling for 3 minutes or put into alcohol 70 per cent for 10 minutes (wired).
3. Applicators, pledgets, small squares, and towels: Keep sterile in covered jars in which they have been sterilized in autoclave.
4. Lifting forceps: Keep sterile in liquor cresolis compositus solution 5 per cent.

To set up sterile tray
1. Lift sterile towel with lifting forceps, and with second pair of forceps open and spread over tray. The edge of the tray must be completely covered. Use second towel if first towel is not sufficiently large to do this.
2. With lifting forceps place sterilized articles as indicated in diagram.
3. Cover with a sterile towel and carry to bedside.

To set up a tray a part of which is sterile
1. Lift sterile towel with lifting forceps, open, and spread over one half of tray. Let the free end of the towel hang from the tray.
2. With the lifting forceps place the sterilized articles as indicated in the diagram.
3. With the lifting forceps turn back the free end of the towel over the set-up tray.
4. Arrange the unsterile articles as indicated in the diagram.

Care of tubing and stopcocks
1. Following use, drop immediately into cold water. As soon as possible rinse thoroughly by forcing water through by means of a syringe. Use a small brush for cleaning stopcocks.
2. Boil in water for 5 minutes or leave in liquor cresolis compositus solution 1 per cent for 15 minutes.
3. Rinse and dry the tubing by stripping. Complete the drying by forcing air through by means of a rubber bulb.

Care of needles
1. Following use, wash immediately in cold water.
2. Scrub with Bon Ami. (Use cork and scrub from base to point.)
3. Dip stillete in Bon Ami, insert in the needle and draw back and fourth several times to polish calibre of needle. Force water through with bulb.
4. Dry the needles thoroughly.
5. Fill the syringe with ether and expel through the needle several times.
6. With rubber bulb blow out every drop of fluid. When perfectly dry replace the wire, which has been dipped into liquid albolene.

Venepuncture

Aim

1. To collect blood for diagnostic purposes.
2. To withdraw blood from the circulation.

Preparation of tray

a. Cover one-half of tray with sterile towel; on this place the following sterile articles:

1. 4 pledgets.
2. 20 cc. syringe.
3. 1 towel.
4. Medicine glass containing alcohol 70 per cent.
5. 2 needles (venepuncture).

Sterile		Unsterile	
3	5	11	10
2			9
1	4	6-7-8	

b. Fold the other half of towel over the set-up tray.
c. On the other half of tray place the following unsterile articles:

6. Small rubber sheet.
7. Towel.
8. Tourniquet (rubber tubing ¼-½ inch diameter).
9. Kidney basin.
10. Bottle with lifting forceps in liquor cresolis compositus solution 5 per cent.
11. Medicine glass or receptacle containing cold water for used needles.

Preparation of patient's arm

1. Expose arm by removing sleeve of gown.
2. Place rubber sheet and unsterile towel under the exposed arm.
3. Place tourniquet about 1-1½ inches above elbow.
4. Sterilize the skin at the point of insertion of needle (about 4 inches square) by cleansing with pledge of cotton dipped into alcohol. Dry surface with a dry pledget.
5. Fasten the tourniquet as tightly as required to make the veins stand out prominently.

Procedure

1. When blood is to be collected for special laboratory purposes, a test tube with sodium oxalate is used.
2. The needle is attached to a 20 cc. syringe and inserted in the vein.
3. When the amount of blood required is obtained, the tourniquet is released, the needle withdrawn, and pressure with a sponge applied over the puncture.
4. If blood is collected for a Wasserman, Wasserman tube is used. The technique is the same as above.

Typhoid Vaccine
(Foreign Protein Therapy)

Aim

1. To introduce a foreign protein and stimulate production of antibodies.

Preparation of tray

a. Cover one-half of tray with sterile towel; on this place the following sterile articles:

1. 4 cotton pledgets.
2. 2 small squares.
3. Towel.
4. 2 venepuncture needles.
5. Paris syringe—20 cc.
6. Medicine glass.
7. Tuberculin syringe.

Sterile			Unsterile		
1		6	8		6
2	5			7	4
3	4	7	9	5	2
				3	1

b. Fold the other half of the towel over the set-up tray.

c. On the other half of tray place the following unsterile articles:
1. Small rubber sheet.
2. Small hand towel.
3. Tourniquet (rubber tubing ¼-½ inch in diameter).
4. Dressing basin.
5. Bottle with lifting forceps.
6. Alcohol for hands.
7. Small bottle of 50 per cent alcohol.
8. Flask of physiological salt solution.
9. Typhoid vaccine.

Preparation of patient's arm

1. The preparation of the arm of the patient is the same as for a venepuncture.
2. At the bedside of the patient, the doctor prepares the vaccine and the physiological salt solution and draws the prepared solution into the syringe ready for use.
3. The care of the patient's arm after giving the vaccine is the same as that following a venepuncture.
4. Typhoid vaccine is given most frequently subcutaneously. The technique is the same as that of any hypodermic injection.

The P. S. P. Test

Aim

1. Phenolsulphonephthalein is a dye that when injected into the body tissues is excreted by the kidneys. By injecting a definite amount and estimating the amount excreted within a certain time, the function of the kidney is tested.

Procedure

1. Have patient empty bladder immediately before injection.

2. Give hypodermic injection of 1 cc. salt solution containing mg. 6 of the dye into the lumbar muscles.
3. Have patient drink two glasses of water just after the injection so that he will be able to urinate at the proper time.
4. Collect urine at exactly one hour and 10 minutes and two hours and 10 minutes after injection, in separate bottles. State on request blank the time of injection and time of collecting urine.

Note: Any medication and liquid nourishment that has been ordered, may be given at stated times. But solid food such as three daily trays should be withheld until the last urination.

To Give Neosalvarsan

Aim
1. To assist in introducing the drug under sterile procedure.

Necessary articles

Sterile tray with:
1. 8 cotton pledgets.
2. 2 needles (venepuncture).
3. Medicine glass.
4. Paris syringe.
5. Sterile towel.

Unsterile tray with:
1. Small rubber sheet.
2. Towel.
3. Tourniquet.
4. Kidney basin.
5. Bottle with thumb forceps in creosol.
6. Medicine glasses or receptacle of cold water for used needles.
7. Flask of freshly distilled water.

Sterile		Unsterile	
			5
1			4
	4		3
2		6	
	5		2
3			1
		7	

Method of preparing neosalvarsan
1. Pour 15 cc. of sterile freshly distilled water into the medicine glass.
2. File ampul containing powdered neosalvarsan and add to above.
3. Mix until thoroughly dissolved by drawing into syringe and forcing it out. Keep tip of syringe under solution while mixing to avoid incorporating air into solution.

Spinal Puncture

Aim
1. To withdraw fluid for diagnostic or therapeutic purposes.

Preparation of tray

a. Cover one-half of tray with sterile towel; on this place the following sterile articles:

1. 1 applicator.
2. 5 cotton pledgets.
3. 3 small squares.
4. 2 sterile towels.
5. 2 spinal puncture needles.
6. Medicine glass with tr. iodine 3.5 per cent.
7. Medicine glass with alcohol 70 per cent.

Sterile		Unsterile	
1	7		13
2	6	14	12
3			11
		8 9	
4	5		10

b. Fold the other half of the towel over the set-up tray.
c. On the other half of the tray place:

8. Small rubber sheet.
9. Kidney basin.
10. Bottle with sterile forceps.
11. Matches for lighting alcohol lamp.
12. Alcohol lamp.
13. Glass (cotton in bottom) holding test tubes numbered 1-2-3.
14. Bottle of alcohol for surgeon's hands.

Preparation of the patient

1. Remove the pillows. Have the patient lie on his side and near the edge of the bed. Flex the body bringing the chin as near the knees as possible. (This position arches the body, brings out the spinal processes, and opens the interspaces between the processes.)
2. Protect the bed with the small rubber sheet. Expose back and paint skin (about 4 inches square), at and above the point of insertion of the needle, using tr. of iodine 3.5 per cent. Remove iodine with alcohol swab. Dry surface with cotton pledgets.
3. Surround the prepared space with sterile towels.

Method of assisting surgeon

1. The surgeon inserts the needle. The nurse, just before the stilette is removed from the needle, selects sterile tube No. 1, removes the plug by touching only the top, flames the rim of the tube and holds ready to collect fluid. Usually about 2 fld. drachms is collected. Tubes 2 and 3 are used in the same way if three tubes are used.
2. As the surgeon withdraws the needle, the nurse has the collodion and swab ready. The wound is sealed with the collodion. No dressing is used.
3. The patient is instructed to stay in bed and to lie without a pillow or with a small one for several hours.

Transfusion

Aim

1. To stimulate bone marrow to greater activity.
2. To replace body fluid lost through hemorrhage.

Procedure

1. Blood is given intravenously by gravity.

Preparation of trays

Sterile				Unsterile		
1	5	14	12			4
2		13	11	7		
3	6				6	3
4			10	8		2
7		8	9		5	1

1. 2 applicators.
2. 8 small squares.
3. 8 thumb sponges.
4. 4 sterile towels.
5. 4 venepuncture needles:
   a. 2 heavy base.
   b. 2 small base.
6. 20 cc. Paris syringe.
7. Sterile fluff.
8. 2 medicine glasses, alcohol, and iodine.
9. Kelly flask.
10. Rubber tubing, 3 feet.
11. Adaptor.
12. Clamp.
13. 1000 cc. flask for collecting blood.
14. Funnel.

1. 2 small rubber sheets.
2. 2 small hand towels.
3. Tourniquet.
4. Dressing basin.
5. Alcohol 70 per cent.
6. Iodine 3½ per cent.
7. Flask of sodium citrate 1½ per cent.
8. Flask of physiological salt.

Preparation of patient and donor

1. If possible, have the beds of the donor and patient in the same room and as near together as convenient.
2. Have a clean stand at each bedside for trays.
3. The arms of donor and patient are prepared exactly the same way as for a venepuncture.
4. Before the blood is withdrawn, the doctor measures the amount of sodium citrate used (about 16 cc. to 100 cc. of blood) into the graduate flask into which the blood is to be withdrawn and prepares the apparatus syringe to be used, so that after the blood is withdrawn it can be injected into the vein of the patient as quickly as possible.

5. The amount of blood withdrawn from the donor varies, the maximum amount being about 500 cc.
6. The method of giving the blood to the patient is the same as that of gravity.
7. The care of the arms after withdrawing and injecting of blood is the same as that following a venepuncture.

LESSON V
STERILE SUPPLIES AND TRAYS, Continued
Hypodermoclysis

Aim
1. To supply fluid to the tissues subcutaneously in:
   a. Hemorrhage.
   b. To stimulate the circulation in shock or collapse.
   c. Postoperative condition.
   d. To dilute the poisons, flush the kidneys, and carry away the poisons in toxemia.

Derivation of the word "hypodermoclysis"
Hypo=beneath.
Derma=skin.
Clysis=to flood.

Solutions usually ordered
1. Physiological salt solution.
2. Lock's solution.

Quantity injected
From 500 to 1000 cc.

Sites of injection
1. Beneath the skin of the abdomen.
2. In the loose tissue at the base of the breasts.
3. In the thighs or buttocks.
4. In the axillary line.

General instructions
1. Be sure that the solution is correct.
2. Have temperature of solution 120°F.
3. Carry out procedure under sterile technique.

Necessary articles
2 medicine glasses for iodine and alcohol.
2 square sponges.
Container, tubing with glass Y connecting tip with two pieces of rubber and clamp.
2 sterile towels.
Applicators with cotton.
Standard.
2 hot water bags and covers.
2 narrow strips of adhesive 6 inches long.
Sterile solution.
2 needles.
Kidney basin.
Cotton for mouth of container.

Nurse's duties

1. Prepare tray and carry to bedside.
2. Prepare the patient and assist the doctor.
   The doctor connects the sterile tubing, etc., disinfects the skin, and inserts the needles.
3. Watch the rate at which the fluid is absorbed.
4. See that the temperature is maintained.
5. Watch patient to avoid exposure and chilling.
6. Watch the patient's color and pulse closely.
7. Place hot water bags near axillae over tubing.
8. Give as ordered: continuous or 2 hours off and 2 hours on.
9. The doctor removes needles. Leave area covered with dry sponge dressing.

Record (in red ink)

1. Hour and treatment.
2. Quantity of fluid.
3. Pulse rate before and after treatment.
4. Any unusual symptoms.
5. By whom performed.

Care of tray after use

1. Clean all articles thoroughly.
2. Inspect articles and replace in perfect condition.
3. Be sure that tubing is not coiled at right angles and that clamps are released.
4. Wrap tray and contaminated articles with large square of muslin and pin securely.
5. Label on the outside as follows:
   "Hypodermoclysis"—double or single.
   Date, floor, and name of nurse.
6. Pin a list of articles on outside of wrapper.

Thoracentesis

Aim

1. To withdraw fluid for diagnostic or therapeutic purposes.

Preparation of trays

a. Cover one-half of tray with sterile towel. On this place the following articles:
   1. 5 sterile applicators.
   2. 4 cotton pledgets.
   3. 4 small squares.
   4. Towel.
   5. Paris syringe, 20 cc.
   6. 2 thoracentesis needles.
   7. Medicine glass.
   8. Hypodermic syringe and needles.

Sterile			Unsterile			
1		10	14	13	10	
2	9			12	7 8	9
6			11	5		
3 5		8			3 4	
4	7		16		1 2	6
			15			

9. Stopcock and cork.
10. Aspirating tube (glass connecting tube inserted) about 12 inches long, with metal tips for connecting with needle and stopcock.
b. Fold the other half of the towel over the set-up tray.
c. On the unsterile half of the tray place the following articles:
1. Small rubber sheet.
2. Kidney basin.
3. Small bottle of alcohol 70 per cent.
4. Iodine 3½ per cent.
5. Bottle with lifting forceps.
6. Collodion.
7. Glass (cotton in bottom) holding two sterile test tubes.
8. Alcohol lamp.
9. Matches.
10. Large (four liter) graduated bottle.
11. Rubber tube about 6 inches long with metal tips for connecting with stopcock and pump.
12. Air pump.
13. Small draw sheet.
14. Adhesive.
15. Bottle of alcohol for disinfecting hands.
16. Camphorated oil (for stimulation if needed).

Preparation of patient

1. Support the patient in sitting posture with back to the side of the bed.
2. Remove the sleeve of the gown on the affected side.
3. Bring gown around to the opposite side and pin. This makes a holder for the rubber sheet and sterile towel.
4. Place the patient's hand on affected side on the opposite shoulder.
5. Cover shoulders with small square sheet.
6. Place small rubber sheet in holder made by pinning gown.
7. At and about the point of insertion of needle (designated by the physician) paint the skin with iodine 3½ per cent. Allow the iodine to dry. Then remove the iodine with alcohol 70 per cent.
8. Dry the surface with a cotton pledge. Place a sterile towel over the rubber sheet.

Method of assisting

1. For diagnostic purpose or when only a small amount of fluid is to be withdrawn:
a. Pour about 4 mils (cc.) of novocaine into the sterile medicine glass. The physician will draw the solution into the hypodermic syringe and anesthetize the area about the point of insertion of thoracentesis needle. He then attaches

the thoracentesis needle to the syringe, inserts into the pleural cavity and withdraws fluid.

    b. Light the alcohol lamp ready to flame the rim of one of the sterile tubes when ready to receive the fluid. A second tube may or may not be used.

    c. As the physician withdraws the needle have a swab and collodion ready with which to seal the wound. A dressing may be used instead.

2. For therapeutic purpose:

    a. The nurse exhausts the air in the graduated bottle by use of air pump (note arrow on nozzle of pump. The arrow on tip attached to bottle must point toward pump.) The physician anesthetizes area about point of insertion of needle with novocaine.

    b. Bring the bottle close to the patient. The physician fastens the needle firmly to the sterile rubber tube, then inserts the needle into the pleural cavity.

    c. When directed by the physician, the nurse opens the valve of the tube leading from the patient, and the fluid will flow slowly into the bottle.

    d. Close the wound in the same manner as directed in the preceding method.

Abdominal Paracentesis

Aim

1. To withdraw fluid for diagnostic or therapeutic purposes.

Preparation of trays

    a. Cover one-half of tray with sterile towel. On this place the following articles:

1. 5 applicators.
2. 5 pledgets.
3. 4 small squares.
4. Sterile towel.
5. Sterile fluff.
6. Sterile abdominal pad.
7. Small scalpel.
8. Trocar, medium size.
9. Medicine glass.
10. Hypodermic syringe with needle.
11. Rubber tubing, 12 inches.
12. Scalpel to make skin incision.

Sterile			Unsterile		
1	6	8	13	12	5
2	7	10	14	8 9	
3			6	7	
4	5	11	3	4	11
9	12		1	2	10

    b. Fold the other half of the towel over the set-up tray.

    c. On the other half of the tray place the following articles:

1. Small rubber sheet.
2. Dressing basin.
3. Iodine 3½ per cent.

4. Small bottle of alcohol 70 per cent.
5. Bottle with lifting forceps.
6. Novocaine 1 per cent.
7. Collodion.
8. Glass (cotton in bottom) holding two sterile test tubes.
9. Alcohol lamp.
10. Matches.
11. Large flat basin to collect fluid.
12. Draw sheet.
13. Adhesive.
14. Bottle of alcohol for disinfecting hands.
   Have ready at the bedside a large pail for large amount of fluid, or if patient sits in chair fluid may be collected in pail.

Preparation of the patient

1. Have the patient empty bladder. A distended bladder might easily be punctured.
2. Shave, if necessary, an area on lower abdomen (4 to 6 inches square), at and about the point of insertion of the trocar.
3. Have the patient sit on a straight backed chair if possible. If not, he may sit either on the side of the bed with legs hanging well over the edge, feet resting on a foot rest or the rungs of a chair. Or he may sit up against pillows at the head of the bed with legs extended straight forward. Bring the gown up well under the arms and fasten at the back.
3. Place a small rubber sheet over the lap well against lower abdomen below prepared skin surface. Paint the skin (shaved surface) with iodine 3½ per cent. Remove iodine with alcohol. Dry surface with cotton pledget.
4. Place sterile towel over rubber sheet.

Method of assisting physician

1. The physician anesthetizes the area about the point of insertion of the trocar, then makes a small incision with the scalpel, and inserts trocar and canula. The nurse has ready the flat basin to collect the fluid. A small amount of fluid is allowed to flow into the basin.
2. The nurse removes the plug from a sterile test tube, flames the rim, and holds it ready to receive the fluid. One or two tubes as requested may be used. The remainder of the fluid or as much as the physician wishes to withdraw is collected in the basin or pan.
3. As the fluid is being withdrawn, the nurse must observe the patient closely for symptoms of collapse.
4. As the physician withdraws the trocar, the nurse has ready a cotton pledget for cleansing the wound. If wound remains

dry, it may be sealed with collodion. If fluid yet oozes from the wound, a dressing fluff and abdominal pad must be used and held in place with an abdominal binder.

5. The patient is instructed to lie quietly in bed for several hours following the treatment.

LESSON VI
STERILE FOMENTATIONS

Aim

1. To relieve pain.
2. To relieve inflammation.
3. To relieve congestion and promote suppuration.

General instructions

1. Keep dressings hot.
2. Apply as hot as can be comfortably borne.
3. Avoid burning the patient.
4. Avoid chilling the part before, during, or after the treatment.
5. Use aseptic technique.

Necessary articles

Bath blanket.
Stupe tray with:
    Basin.
    Stupe wringer and sticks.
    Two pieces of flannel (twice the size of the abdomen), one dry and one wet.
    Gauze dressings, dry and wet (size to be determined by size of area to be treated).
    Oiled muslin or waxed paper.
    Binder, triangular bandage, bandage or bath towel, depending on location of dressing.
    2 forceps.
    Safety pins.
    Receptacle for soiled dressings.
    Hot water bag and cover.

Preparation

1. Wash your hands.
2. Place gauze and flannel in stupe wringer and place in basin.
3. Fill basin with water being sure that stupe wringer is well covered.
4. Put forceps in basin.
5. Place basin in the sterilizer or over a flame and boil for 15 minutes. (Be sure that the water in the sterilizer comes up over the basin, otherwise the articles will not be sterile.)
6. If a solution other than water is used, the stupe wringer is placed in basin with solution and boiled over gas burner. Prepare the hot water bottle.
7. Remove basin, wring dressings and flannel dry with stupe wringer.
8. Pour out water and place stupe wringer with flannel and forceps in basin.

9. Cover with oiled muslin or waxed paper and dry flannel.
10. Arrange all articles on the tray and carry to the bedside.

Procedure

1. Screen the patient.
2. Cover patient to avoid chilling.
3. Prepare articles ready for use before exposing area.
4. Remove outer dressings with a third forceps or with the hands.
5. Remove soiled dressings with one of the sterile forceps and place in container, paper bag, or newspaper.
6. Replace soiled dressings with one layer of dry sterile gauze.
7. Open wringer, using forceps, shake gauze dressings to incorporate air and apply quickly. Then apply wet flannel.
8. Cover with oiled muslin or waxed paper and then with dry flannel.
9. Adjust binder or bandage to keep dressings in place.
10. Apply hot water bottle to keep dressings hot.
11. Arrange bedclothes.
12. Second fomentation prepared in the same way before the first one is removed.
13. Dressings are usually changed every two hours.
   Note: The dressings that are saturated with drainage are discarded; the others are boiled, washed in soap and water, rinsed, dried, and used again for the same patient. When possible it is desirable to have a tray with the necessary articles for each patient.

Record

1. Time and treatment.
2. Method of application.
3. Drainage, and patient's reaction to the treatment.

LESSON VII
VAGINAL DOUCHE

Aim

1. To cleanse the vagina.
2. To arrest local hemorrhages.
3. To relieve inflammation.

General instructions

1. Avoid burning the patient when giving hot douches by allowing solution to run slowly and with little force.
2. If patient is menstruating, do not give douche unless ordered by doctor.
3. Place the patient in a recumbent position before giving douche.
4. Patient's shoulders should be lower than hips.
5. Have patient remain quiet one hour after giving douche.
6. Have patient void before giving douche.
7. Do not touch point before inserting, nor after removing.
8. Use extreme care if there are stitches in the perineum. Examine douche nozzle for rough edges, and be sure that it is not cracked or broken.
9. Do not permit the patient to insert douche point or to take her own douche.

Types

1. For cleansing and stimulating; solutions usually ordered:
   a. Sterile water.
   b. Physiological salt solution.
   c. Lysol or cresolis compositus solution ½ per cent.
   d. Dram 1 iodine solution to 2 quarts water or as ordered.
   e. Potassium permanganate solution as ordered.
   f. Bichloride of mercury as ordered.
2. For reducing inflammation and arresting hemorrhage; solution usually ordered:
   a. Physiological salt solution.
   b. Sterile water.

Temperature of solution

1. For cleansing, 105° F.
2. For inflammation, 115° F.
3. For hemorrhage, 120° F.

Quantity generally used

1. Two or three quarts.

Position of patient

2. Dorsal recumbent.

Necessary articles

Standard.

Douche can with tubing.
Sterile dressing towel.
2 sterile cotton balls.
Douche pan.
Sterile perineal pad.
Kidney basin.
Sterile thermometer.
Douche point.
Large sheet.
Rubber protector.
Bed-pan cover (2).
Sterile graduate, 1000 cc.
Sterile forceps.

Preparation

1. Sterilize douche can, tubing, kidney basin, forceps, douche point, and graduate, by boiling ten minutes.
2. Prepare solution ordered. Heat by allowing can to stand in sterilizer.

Procedure

1. Screen patient and place standard.
2. Carry other articles to bedside, also douche pan, covered with sterile dressing towel which covers can, on tray.
3. Hang can covered with sterile dressing towel on standard.
4. Fanfold all bedding to the foot of the bed and replace by a large sheet.
5. Drape the patient as for pelvic examination.
6. Place the protector and bed-pan cover under buttocks.
7. Place douche pan.
8. Allow solution to run through tubing into pan until warm.
9. Cleanse vulva with jet from tubing using ⅓ of solution.
10. Clamp off tubing and connect douche point.
11. Insert point gently downward and backward into vagina.
12. Remove point before all solution has left can.
13. Disconnect point and replace in kidney basin. Dry patient with cotton balls.
14. Place perineal pad and straighten bed.
15. Boil douche point after using.

Record

1. Hour and treatment.
2. Kind and strength of solution.
3. Character of return flow.
    Note: If a cleansing instead of aseptic douche, follow the foregoing procedure using the following articles: clean instead of sterile towel, solution, perineal pad, and cotton balls. If the can is not contaminated, it can be used for other cleansing douches.

LESSON VIII

CATHETERIZATION AND BLADDER IRRIGATION

Female Catheterization

Aim

1. To remove urine from the bladder.

General instructions

1. Never catheterize without an order.
2. Use every known means to get patient to void first unless special orders are given following some operation or treatment.
3. Use glass catheters at all times except when rubber catheters are indicated or ordered.
4. Remember there is great danger of infection; use sterile technique.

Necessary articles

Tray with:
2 glass catheters with small rubber tubing 2 inches long.
Catheter basin with cover.
1 dressing towel to cover tray.
2 small sterile sponges.
12 sterile cotton balls.
2 enamel dressing bowls with enamel covers.
Large sheet for draping.
Rubber protector.
Bed-pan cover.
Hemostat.
Sterile boric acid solution.
Flashlight or extension light.
2 kidney basins (large and small).

Preparation

1. After water is actually boiling, leave catheter basin, catheters, hemostat, dressing bowls and covers in sterilizer for five minutes.
2. Remove dressing bowls from sterilizer with forceps and place on tray.
3. Drop sterile cotton balls into one bowl.
4. Pour enough warm, sterile, boric acid solution over sterile cotton balls to saturate.
5. Place covers on dressing bowls.
6. Place catheter basin containing catheters and hemostat on the tray. Place forceps with handle away from round end of catheters.
7. Drop two small sterile sponges into catheter basin and cover.
8. Place kidney basins on the tray.

9. Place large sheet, rubber protector, and bed-pan cover on the tray.
10. Cover tray with dressing towel and carry to bedside.

Procedure

1. Screen the patient.
2. Drape patient as for pelvic examination.
3. Cover rubber protector with bed-pan cover and place under buttocks.
4. Place tray on foot of bed or on stand at foot of bed.
5. Place flashlight or extension light.
6. Remove the towel.
7. Wash hands thoroughly.
8. Remove enamel covers.
9. Place empty dressing bowl in position to receive urine.
10. Place smaller kidney basin in position to receive pledgets.
11. Place larger kidney basin where it can be used if there is an unusual amount of urine.
12. Place small sterile sponges on each side of labia.
13. Part labia with thumb and forefinger of the left hand to expose meatus.
14. Keep this hand in place throughout procedure.
15. Using hemostat, cotton balls, and sterile boric acid solution, cleanse the area between the labia majora.
16. Beginning at the top, make one downward stroke with each ball.
17. Cleanse with ten cotton balls, and place the eleventh in the mouth of the vagina.
18. Pick up catheter by the rubber. Inspect catheter.
19. Hold with curved part down; insert very gently into the meatus. Gradually, turn the catheter as it enters.
20. After urine begins to run slowly, pinch tubing and withdraw the catheter gently.
21. Touch the meatus with the last cotton ball.
22. Remove the cotton from the vagina.
23. Remove all articles and make patient comfortable.

Care of articles after use

1. Wash immediately with cold water.
2. Boil all articles that are contaminated.
3. Dry thoroughly and replace on tray.
4. Leave tray clean and complete.
5. Replace tray on shelf.

Record (in red ink)

1. Hour and treatment.
2. Amount and color of urine.
3. Character and odor.

To secure sterile specimen
1. Add sterile specimen bottle with cover to necessary articles.

To secure specimen for culture
1. Culture tube.
2. Alcohol lamp and matches if tube is not covered with sterile protector.

Male Catheterization

Nurse's duties
1. The nurse prepares the tray, calls the interne, carries tray to bedside, and screens the patient.
2. After catheterization the nurse removes the tray, measures the urine, and records catheterization.

Necessary articles
2 catheters (wax and hard or soft rubber).
Catheter basin.
Dressing bowls with covers, one for boric acid solution and one to receive the urine.
2 sterile towels.
4 cotton balls, 2 on the tray and 2 in solution.
Kidney basin.
Sterile lubricant, usually vaseline, on sterile sponge.

Preparation
1. Soak catheters of hard rubber or wax in 1-1000 bichloride solution in catheter basin for ½ hour.
2. Rinse with sterile water.
3. If rubber catheters are used, boil.
4. Boil dressing bowls and kidney basin.
5. Set up tray with sterile towels, one under and one over articles.

Bladder Irrigation

Aim
1. To cleanse bladder.
2. To reduce inflammation.

General instructions
1. See procedure for catheterization.
2. Do not over-distend bladder with cleansing solution.
3. Have the solution the correct temperature.
4. If a medication is used after irrigation, warm by setting medicine glass in basin of hot water.

Solutions usually ordered
1. Boric acid.
2. Physiological salt solution.

3. Potassium permanganate 1-1000.
4. Silver nitrate 1-1000.
5. Protargol 1-1000.

Temperature of solution
1. From 105° to 108° F.

Amount of solution
1. From 1 to 2 quarts.

Position of Patient
1. Dorsal recumbent position.

Necessary articles
In addition to articles for catheterization:
Sterile glass funnel.
Connecting tip.
Rubber tubing on funnel.
Sterile thermometer.
Small tubing on glass catheter, 2 inches.

Procedure
1. Catheterize patient and without withdrawing catheter, attach connecting tip with rubber tubing and funnel to small rubber tip on catheter.
2. Pour in solution slowly, six to eight ounces.
3. Invert funnel before it is empty and siphon two-thirds of the amount given.
4. Pour in four to five ounces and siphon.
5. Repeat until solution returns clean, using from one to two quarts.

Record (in red ink)
1. Hour.
2. Amount of urine withdrawn.
3. Amount and strength of solution used.
4. Character of return flow.

Care of articles after use
1. Sterilize, clean, and leave dry. Replace tray on shelf with equipment complete.

LESSON IX

The Sponge Bath

Aim

1. To improve the circulation and respiration.
2. To increase elimination.
3. To relieve restlessness and to make the patient more comfortable.
4. To lower the temperature.

General instructions

1. Do not allow the patient to be in a draught.
2. Encourage patient to breathe deeply during the treatment.
3. Give plenty of cool water unless contraindicated.
4. Apply cold to the head.
5. Apply heat to the feet to prevent chilling and to counterbalance temperature between central and peripheral portions of the body.
6. Use friction for the same reason as for the application of heat to the feet.
7. During any of the treatments, watch for evidence of shock:
   a. Weak, irregular pulse.
   b. Pallor about the mouth.
   c. Cyanosis of finger nails.
   d. Slow and shallow respirations.
8. In case of shock, stop treatment, apply external heat, and report condition to the head nurse at once.
9. Mop water from the bed at intervals during sponge.
10. Sponge is given whenever the temperature is 102.6° F. or whenever ordered.

Necessary articles

Large rubber sheet (length of mattress).
Cotton draw sheet.
Hot water bag and cover.
Ice bag and cover or ice compresses.
Foot tub ½ full of water at temperature ordered, usually 78-85° F. (may begin with water at 85° and gradually lower to 75°).
Bath thermometer.
Cracked ice.
Bath blanket.
Towels (face and bath).
2 large loose sponges of gauze (1 yd.).

Procedure

1. Fanfold bed covers to the foot of the bed.
2. Replace covers with the bath blanket.

3. Pass the rubber sheet covered with draw sheet under the patient.
4. Remove the gown.
5. Place ice bag to the head and hot water bag to the feet.
6. Give friction for 2 or 3 minutes over the entire body.
7. Sponge face and dry with face towel.
8. Fold back blanket, exposing ½ of body from neck to foot.
9. Then proceed to sponge using long, even strokes.
10. Sponge with one hand, giving friction with the other.
11. Begin high on neck (hair line), sponge down over shoulder and outer surface of arm.
12. Turn sponge in hand, begin at hair line, and sponge over shoulder and inner arm.
13. Change sponge; beginning at the axilla sponge down side and over outer surface of thigh to foot.
14. Turn sponge in hand, begin at axilla and sponge over chest and abdomen and inner surface of thigh to foot.
15. Continue, changing sponge each second stroke until exposed surface of body has been covered. Continue for 7-8 minutes.
16. Then fold bath blanket over sponged surface, exposing other half of the body.
17. Proceed in the same way for 7-8 minutes.
18. Cover the patient with the bath blanket and turn on the side to expose back.
19. Begin at hair line and sponge length of back to the feet. Continue for about 6 minutes.
20. Turn patient on back and leave wrapped in wet blanket and sheet for 10 minutes.

To remove from the bath

1. Roll sheet and rubber sheet close to the back. Dry the back if necessary then turn on to the dry bed and quickly remove the rubber and sheet.
2. Complete the drying of the body if necessary.
3. An alcohol sponge may be given if it adds to the patient's comfort.
4. Replace the gown.
5. Pull up the covers and remove the bath blanket.

Changes to expect

1. The patient is usually much more comfortable and may fall asleep.
2. The respirations are fuller and deeper. The pulse is usually 5-10 beats per minute slower and more regular both as to rhythm and force.
3. The temperature, pulse, and respirations should be taken ½ hour after the completion of the bath.

Record
1. Hour and treatment.
2. Duration and temperature of sponge.
3. Condition of patient.
4. Temperature after bath.

The Alcohol Sponge

Aim
1. To improve the circulation and respiration.
2. To increase elimination.
3. To relieve restlessness and to make the patient more comfortable.
4. To lower the temperature.

General instructions
1. Given when you wish to disturb the patient as little as possible.
2. See "The Sponge Bath."

Necessary articles

3 bath towels.
1 bath blanket.
Ice bag and cover.
Hot water bag and cover.
Gauze sponge.
Alcohol 25 per cent, 1 pint.

Procedure
1. Fanfold the covers to the foot of the bed.
2. Replace covers with the bath blanket.
3. Remove the gown.
4. Place one bath towel under one arm and close to and under the side.
5. Place the second towel under the other side.
6. Place the third towel under the legs and feet bringing it well up under the hips.
7. Place the ice bag at the head and a hot water bag at the feet.
8. Expose ½ of the body from the neck to the feet and sponge in the same way as in the procedure for the sponge bath except that it is necessary to press the solution from the sponge so that none will drip on the bed.
9. Continue until entire anterior surface is covered.
10. Do not turn the patient but sponge the back by moistening the palms of the hands in the solution and slipping them under the back.
11. The duration of the bath is 20 minutes.
12. Remove the bath towels.
13. Dry the skin and make up the bed as usual.

14. If the bath has been given to lower the temperature, the temperature should be taken ½ hour after the completion of the bath.

Record

1. Hour and treatment.
2. Any unusual symptoms which may occur.
3. Temperature after bath.

LESSON X
SEDATIVE TREATMENTS
The Sedative Pack

Aim
1. For insomnia.
2. For the treatment of drug addicts.
3. For disorders of the nervous system.

Necessary articles

Foot tub ½ full of water at 85°.
Bath thermometer.
2 small sheets.
2 bath blankets.
Large rubber sheet.
Hot water bag and cover.
Ice bag and cover.
1 face towel.
1 bath towel.

Procedure
1. Fanfold the covers to the foot of the bed.
2. Replace covers with the bath blanket.
3. Pass the rubber sheet covered with the bath blanket under the patient.
4. Remove the gown.
5. Place the ice bag at the head and the hot water bag at the feet.
6. Fanfold one small sheet lengthwise, and the other one crosswise.
7. Place in the tub of water; remove and wring dry.
8. Place the one folded lengthwise under the patient and the one folded crosswise over the patient underneath the bath blanket.
9. Give friction for two or three minutes through the wet sheet and underneath the bath blanket.
10. Tuck blankets snugly around the patient.
11. Use another blanket if needed for warmth.
12. Continue pack for time ordered, one hour or longer.
13. If the patient goes to sleep in the pack do not disturb.

To remove the pack
1. Have a hot drink ready for the patient.
2. Remove the wet sheets disturbing the patient as little as possible and put on a warm gown.
3. Give hot drink and leave patient. Be sure that the room is well ventilated and warm.

Record
1. Hour and treatment.
2. Duration and temperature of pack.
3. Condition of the patient.

The Sitz Bath

Aim

1. To relieve tenesmus in uterine and renal colic.
2. To relax the sphincter of the bladder and overcome retention of urine.
3. To relieve sciatica.
4. To relieve pain, congestion, and inflammation in the organs of the pelvis.
5. To restore the menstrual function.
6. To relieve painful hemorrhoids.

Necessary articles

Sitz tub.
Foot tub.
3 blankets.
Ice cap or cold compress.
Thermometer.
3 bath towels.
Water in sitz tub 106° F. to 120° F.
Water in foot tub 110° F. to 120° F.

Procedure

1. Have the bathroom warm.
2. Cover chair with bath blanket and bath towel.
3. Prepare the tubs of water, one at 106° F. and one at 110° F. (see above).
4. Place a bath towel over the edge of the tub.
5. Take patient to the bathroom unless tub is portable.
6. Remove gown and kimona.
7. Drape other bath blanket around shoulders with open side at the back.
8. Pin blanket at the neck.
9. Place cold applications to head.
10. Have patient sit in the sitz tub with feet in foot tub.
11. Be sure that the patient is immersed from the waist to well below thighs.
12. Cover limbs and feet with second blanket, being sure that the baths are enclosed in the blankets.
13. Duration of bath, 3 to 10 minutes, or as long as ordered.
14. Increase temperature of water in tubs up to 120° F. or as hot as patient can stand it.
15. Watch pulse and general condition of patient.
16. When bath is completed, assist the patient from the tub and dry the external genitals and thighs.
17. Put on slippers.
18. Have her sit on the chair and put on her kimona as you remove the bath blanket.

19. Take the patient back to her room and put her to bed.
20. Clean the tubs and leave room in perfect order.

Record

1. Hour and treatment.
2. Duration of treatment.
3. Temperature of water.
4. Patient's reaction to the treatment.

LESSON XI
THE HOT PACK

Aim
1. To induce perspiration.
2. To relieve edema.
3. To eliminate waste products.

General instructions
1. Apply cold to the head and keep the feet warm to prevent the dilatation and congestion of the cerebral blood vessels.
2. Avoid burning the patient.
3. Watch for symptoms of heat prostration such as soft, weak, or irregular pulse, sighing respirations, flushed face, etc.
4. Avoid exposing the patient while covers are being removed.
5. Give plenty of fluids (preferably hot) unless liquids are restricted.
6. Work quickly when putting on the steamed blankets. If necessary, use towels for handling.

Necessary articles
4 wool blankets (1 old, thin one).
3 cotton blankets.
Large rubber sheet (mackintosh).
Rubber draw sheet.
Ice bag and cover.
Hot water bag and cover.
Towels (1 face and 1 bath).
Foot tub or bath basin.
Tray containing a drink such as lemonade, tea, etc., preferably hot, if liquids are not restricted.
Bottle of alcohol as for back rub.

Procedure
1. To prepare the blankets:
   a. Roll the large rubber sheet between 2 wool blankets.
   b. Place the thin, old one on top.
   c. Fold and place on radiator, in blanket warmer, or with hot water bags, to be warmed.
   d. Warm third wool blanket also.
   e. Fanfold both sides of first cotton blanket lengthwise in thirds to center, double over, and roll.
   f. Fold second cotton blanket end to end, in half, then fold back edges to meet center fold.
   g. Fold third cotton blanket the same as the second cotton blanket.

h. Wet the 3 rolled blankets and wring as dry as possible.

i. Place wet blankets over inverted foot tub or basin in tray of utensil sterilizer. (Basin in sterilizer used to prevent the blankets from touching the water.)

j. Invert foot tub over top of sterilizer. Place the folded smaller sheet on top of tub so that both will be warmed.

k. Steam blankets in sterilizer for 20 or 30 minutes.

2. To prepare the patient:

a. Fanfold the covers to the foot of the bed, covering the patient at the same time with the warmed wool blanket.

b. Put the rolled blankets and rubber sheet under the patient, the old, thin, wool blanket next to patient.

c. Remove the gown.

d. Wrap patient well in the old wool blanket. (This is to prevent burning as the wet blankets must not touch the skin.)

e. Place the ice bag at the head and the hot water bag at the feet.

3. To give the pack:

a. Line the foot tub with the small rubber draw sheet. Into this place the blankets from the sterilizer, the one folded lengthwise last.

b. Carry well covered to the bedside.

c. Take and record pulse.

d. Place lengthwise folded blanket under the patient, tucking well around the body and high on the shoulder.

e. Place second and third blankets on top of patient, tucking in well around the body.

f. Bring the rubber sheet up around the body.

g. Place rubber draw sheet over all and tuck snugly under at the sides.

h. Bring the dry wool blanket down well under the sides.

i. Draw up the the covers to give greater warmth.

j. Place face towel under patient's chin.

k. Take pulse frequently. Do not leave the patient while in the pack.

l. The patient remains in the pack as long as ordered, usually 20 minutes after sweating begins.

4. To remove the pack:

a. Fanfold covers to the foot of the bed.

b. Remove wet blankets and rubber sheets, leaving the patient between dry blankets. *Do not* expose the patient while removing the blankets.

c. After 30 minutes or 1 hour, dry the patient, give alcohol rub, and remove the wool blankets.

d. Replace the gown.

Record
1. Hour and treatment.
2. Duration of the pack.
3. Effects produced.
4. Any unusual symptoms that may occur.

LESSON XII

TEST MEALS, LAVAGE, AND GAVAGE

Lavage

Aim
1. To wash the stomach.
2. To remove poisons and irritating matter.
3. To relieve nausea.

General instructions
1. Gain the confidence of the patient.
2. When inserting the stomach tube, do not use force, and avoid striking the posterior wall of the pharynx.
3. When pouring the fluid, do not allow the funnel to become empty.
4. Discontinue the treatment at once if blood appears during the siphonage.
5. All lavages are done by the doctor. The nurse assists the doctor.

Solutions usually ordered
1. Sodium bicarbonate.
2. Magnesium sulphate.
3. Physiological saline solution.
4. Rain water.

Temperature of solution
1. From 95° to 105° F.

Quantity of solution
1. From 1 to 4 quarts.

Position of patient
1. Sitting up in bed or chair.
2. Semi-recumbent.

Necessary articles
Tray set up with:
Stomach tube with funnel in basin of ice.
Two face towels.
Kidney basin.
White enamel pitcher.
Small rubber sheet, Kelly pad, or rubber apron.
Pail or foot tub.
Solution.
Cotton draw sheet.

Procedure
1. Set up tray and carry necessary articles to the bedside.

2. Cover rubber sheet with cotton draw sheet, turning back over the edges of rubber, and place it about the patient's neck.
3. Place tub on the floor near the patient.
4. Have the head of the patient supported and insert the tube gently.
5. The tube is usually inserted to the graduated mark, or about 16 inches.
6. Urge the patient to breathe deeply and swallow frequently.
7. Never use force.
8. Pour the solution into the funnel, holding the funnel not too high above the patient's head. Continue until a pint has been introduced into the stomach. Then lower the tube over the pail or tub and siphon.
9. Repeat in accordance with the doctor's orders, or until the water returns clear.
10. When removing tube, pinch it tightly so that any water in the tube may not drop back into the trachea.
11. Replace tray on shelf, clean, and complete.

Record

1. Time and treatment given with kind and amount of solution.
2. Character of solution first returned.
3. Any abnormal conditions present.
4. By whom performed.
   Note: The procedure is written in the above way so that the student will know how a tube is passed as well as be able to assist the doctor.

Ewald, Hawdek, and Fatty Meals

N. P. B. A. Hospital

Patient is to report at 7:00 A. M. without breakfast on morning of examination. Nurse in receiving room will take patient to second floor dressing room and notify head nurse, who sees that Ewald test meal is given at 7:15. Chart time of serving both at central desk and on patient's chart. This is done by the diet nurse. Gastric expression at 8:30, Hawdek to be given at 8:15. If the Ewald meal has been ordered, Hawdek is not given until after the gastric expression. Patient will report at 2:30 without dinner for x-ray examination.

Doctors will write patient's name in appointment book at time of making appointment and indicate whether Ewald or Hawdek or both are to be given.

Ewald test meal: 2 slices of soft bread without crust, 350 cc. of cold water.

Hawdek meal: standard x-ray meal (gm. 30 barium sulphate given in cream of wheat served hot with milk and sugar (no cream).

Fatty meal for gall bladder: 3 egg yolks well beaten, mixed with half a glass of cream.

Gastric Expression

Aim

1. To aid diagnosis by determining:
   a. Motor function of stomach.
   b. Reaction of gastric juice.

General instructions

1. Give meal on an empty stomach.
2. See that patient does not take anything by mouth until meal is removed.
3. Caution patient to masticate slowly and thoroughly.
4. Remove promptly at time desired.
5. All expressions of test meals are done by doctor.
6. The nurse prepares the tray, containing:
   a. Stomach tube in basin of ice.
   b. Politzer bag.
   c. Kidney basin.
   d. Two face towels.
   e. Small rubber sheet or rubber apron.
   f. Conical specimen glass.
   g. Cotton draw sheet.
7. When removing meal, the same precautions are used as for stomach lavage.
8. The nurse assists the doctor as for stomach lavage.

Type of test meals

1. Ewald's test meal:
   a. Two slices of dry toast.
   b. Eight ounces of clear tea.
   c. Remove in one hour, or as ordered.
2. Boa's test meal:
   a. Six ounces of strained oatmeal gruel.
   b. Remove in one hour.
3. Motor meal:
   a. A dinner served of foods that have a great deal of cellulose, such as vegetables with fibre: turnips, cabbage, etc.
   b. Fruits with skins, etc.
   c. Small serving of meat.
   d. Remove in seven hours.

Procedure

1. Prepare patient and pass the tube as in lavage.
2. Expel the air from the bulb; attach to tube; it must be air tight.
3. When the bulb is fully expanded, detach, empty contents

into specimen glass and repeat until all contents are removed.

4. Send the specimen to the laboratory with the request blank.

Record

1. Hour and kind of test meal given.
2. Amount, character, odor, and color of the return.
3. Hour test meal was removed and sent to the laboratory.
4. By whom performed.

Fractional Gastric Expression

Aim

1. To determine the curve of hydrochloric acid in the stomach after an Ewald meal.

Necessary articles

Tray with:
Duodenal tube in dressing bowl of ice.
6 large size test tubes (in a container so that they stand upright).
Litmus paper (red and blue).
Luer or triumph syringe.
Kidney basin.
Rubber band or small forceps.
Articles for preparation of patient same as for gastric expression.

Procedure

1. Nurse prepares the tray and assists the doctor.
2. The patient is given no food before the first expression.
3. The duodenal tube is passed the same as in the other type of gastric expression.
4. The specimen is obtained by aspirating with the syringe.
5. After the first specimen the patient is given an Ewald meal or a meal as ordered by the doctor.
6. The remaining specimens (usually 6 in all) are expressed at intervals of 15 minutes.
7. The tube is kept in the patient's throat and clamped off between specimens with a forceps or rubber band.
8. Send specimens to laboratory with a request blank.

Record

1. Hour and kind of expression.
2. Specimen to the laboratory.

Duodenal Catheterization

Aim

1. To determine whether or not there is a free flow of bile and whether the bile is normal or pathological.
2. For lavage of duodenum with magnesium sulphate or other preparations affecting the bile duct.

Necessary articles

1. Same as for fractional gastric expression.

Procedure

1. Nurse prepares tray and assists doctor.
2. The tube is swallowed by the patient until it is well within the duodenum.
3. Evidences:
   a. A resistance tuck when the tube is pulled.
   b. Appearance of yellow bile with alkaline reaction upon aspiration.
4. Have patient lie on side of bed and elevate hips by placing 3 pillows under them. Remove pillows under head.
5. Proceed as for fractional gastric expression.

Gavage

Aim

1. To introduce food into the stomach when the patient cannot or will not take food in the usual manner.

Necessary articles

Same as for gastric lavage tray.
Graduate with six to eight ounces of prepared food, 105° F., according to the doctor's orders.

Procedure

1. Prepare the patient as for lavage.
2. Introduce the tube as for lavage.
3. Pinch the tube and wait a few seconds before introducing the food.
4. Note respiration.
5. Pour the liquid into the funnel slowly, and at the side.
6. Pinch the tube, withdraw it gently but quickly.
7. Have the patient remain quiet after the treatment.

Record

1. Hour of feeding.
2. Preparation of food given and amount.
3. Result.
4. By whom performed.

Nasal Gavage

Aim

1. To introduce food into the stomach with as little effort to the patient as possible:
   a. When patient is in a weakened condition and cannot swallow food.

b. Operations, carcinoma of tongue, cleft palate, fracture of the jaw, etc.
c. Tetanus, meningitis.
d. Irritable and violent patients.
e. Weak infants.

General instructions

1. Be sure that the catheter is in the esophagus and not in the mouth or larynx.
2. Watch breathing and color of patient while inserting the tube.
3. If obstruction is met, withdraw the tube and insert in the other nostril.

Necessary articles

Medium sized rubber catheter.
Small glass funnel attached.
Lubricant.
Graduate with food same as for gavage, temperature 100° F.
Kidney basin.
Rubber protector.
Face towel.
Safety pin.

Procedure

1. Carry the tray to the bedside.
2. Have patient lying down with the head turned to one side or sitting up with the head tilted forward.
3. Cover rubber protector with face towel and fasten around the neck.
4. Lubricate, then insert catheter, directing toward the septum of the nose so that about 4 inches is passed into the esophagus.
5. Wait until normal breathing is established before pouring in the liquid.
6. Pour in only a few drops at first.
7. When all the fluid has left the funnel, pinch the catheter and quickly withdraw.

Record

1. Hour and treatment.
2. Character and quantity of food given.
3. Any unusual symptoms that may occur.

LESSON XIII

THE CARE OF THE ISOLATED PATIENT

The Care of the Isolated Patient

University Hospital

Complete isolation is

1. Isolation in a separate room, or
2. Isolation by means of screens placed about the lower two-thirds of the bed, preferably about the entire bed.
3. Isolation by removal of the bed to such a position that its center stands at least 10 feet from the center of any adjacent bed.

Visitors

1. Visitors are not permitted in the room or near the patient except when patient is critically ill, and then the visitor must wear a gown.

Gowns

1. Gowns must be worn by examiners, nurses, and attendants while in routine contact with the patient or his bed. This does not mean that it is necessary to wear a gown while palpating a pulse, administering a hypodermic, taking a temperature, etc., but in the performance of these acts one must be careful not to touch the bed or the patient except with the hands and the hands must be washed before touching any other patient or object.
2. There must be a separate set of gowns for use in the care of each patient.
3. Gowns must be changed before going from one patient's room to another.
4. Gowns must not be worn outside the patient's room.
5. Gowns are to be hung with the contaminated side out in the room.
6. Before removal of a gown the hands must be disinfected by washing in basin of lysol solution.
7. After removal of the gown all examiners, attendants, and visitors must scrub their hands thoroughly with soap and water.

Gloves

1. Gloves are to be worn in the care of all acute venereal cases.

Care of linen

1. Secure a striped bag from the laundry or use a clean sheet.
2. Turn back cuff on bag before contaminating hands.
3. As each piece is taken from bed, place in bag.

4. When the linen is collected, wash the hands and close the bag.
5. Tag "boil," and place by the side of clothes hamper.

Care of blankets
1. Air for three days and then send to the laundry.

Care of the mattress
1. Air for three days, turning frequently making it possible for the sun to reach all parts of the mattress, and clean thoroughly.

Care of utensils
1. Before replacing utensils in service room boil them in utensil sterilizer and then scrub with soap and water, rinse, and dry.

Care of rubber goods
1. Immerse in 1 per cent liquor cresolis solution all rubber goods that cannot be boiled for twenty minutes; clean and dry.

Care of dishes
1. Carry to room on tray.
2. Transfer to second tray or table covered with paper napkins, arrange neatly and conveniently.
3. When ready to collect the soiled dishes, carry a clean tray covered with paper napkins to bedside, place soiled dishes on tray, taking care not to contaminate clean tray.
4. Put refuse food in newspaper and put into the waste can.
5. Pour liquids into hopper in service room.
6. Put dishes into tepid water and after water is boiling, boil 15 minutes.
7. The maid removes and washes with other dishes.

To disinfect excreta
1. Chloride of lime 5 per cent, use twice as much of the solution as there is excreta.
   Note: Cases taken to x-ray room or off the floor must be entirely covered with a clean sheet.

The Care of the Isolated Patient

N. P. B. A. Hospital

Aim
1. To prevent transmission of infection from one patient to another.

General instructions
1. Never leave the room with the gown on.
2. Do not fill the hamper bag so full that the string cannot be drawn.
3. Use the isolated hamper bag (square of blue gingham sewed on it).

4. Use a separate laundry bag for blankets, robes, and dark articles.
5. Wear a gown when doing a treatment, examining, or caring for the patient.
6. After caring for the patient, do not touch the face before scrubbing the hands.
7. Do not eat anything the patient has handled.
8. Instruct the patient not to touch the shelf, light button, nurse's gown, or door knob; also not to step on the floor with his bare feet or to handle anything that has dropped to the floor.
9. Observe technique faithfully.
10. Keep service room clean; if contaminated, scrub.

Equipment for the isolated room

1. Bedside table:
   a. Glass and drinking tube.
   b. Soap in a dish.
   c. Face towel.
   d. Bath towel.
   e. Wash cloth.
2. Second table or shelf:
   a. Thermometer.
   b. Alcohol.
   c. Powder.
   d. Bed pan and urinal on lower shelf.
   e. Wash basin.
   f. Mouth-wash cup.
   g. Emesis basin.
3. Table or stand:
   a. Basin of 2 per cent lysol solution.
   b. Two rubber bands in the solution.
4. Hook in the room for the gown.
5. Paper bag pinned to the mattress.
6. Chair.
7. Bed.
8. Additional things that may be added are: tray, sugar, salt and pepper shaker, hot water bottle, and ice cap. (Unnecessary things should not be contaminated; articles not in use should be scrubbed and taken out.)

Procedure

1. Open the bed, making sure that it has a rubber draw sheet on it.
2. Bring in the necessary articles for the care of the patient.
3. Fold the clean gown, so that the contaminated side will be outside.

4. Morning care of the patients:
   a. Collect all the articles necessary before entering the patient's room, as fresh drinking water, linen, medicines, equipment for treatments, water for bathing, ice for ice cap, and dust pan and cloth for cleaning room.
   b. Roll the blue uniform sleeves to the elbows before putting on the isolation gown.
   c. Scrub the clean areas, as the shelf, light button, and door knob.
   d. Take the temperature, give the medicines, do the treatments, give the bath, make the bed, and dust the room. (The maid mops the floor.)
   e. Assemble all the articles to be taken out of the room.
   f. Rinse the hands in lysol.
   g. Remove the gown and put into the laundry bag.
   h. Remove all unnecessary articles to the service room, placing them on a clean piece of paper before they are scrubbed.
   i. Scrub the hands 3 minutes with soap and brush.
   j. Wrap the contaminated articles to be burned in the newspaper on which they are lying and put in the garbage can.

5. Treatment trays:
   a. Place a piece of clean newspaper on the bedside table.
   b. Place the tray on the paper.
   c. Remove corks from solution bottles and pins from sterile dressings.
   d. Put on gown. Doctor or third person may handle articles on tray, keeping them clean; if necessary to contaminate bottle, set it aside and scrub with soap and water before returning to the tray.
   e. Rinse hands in lysol, remove gown, scrub hands, and remove tray from room.

6. Care of dishes:
   a. Place a clean piece of newspaper on the table in the service room.
   b. Remove the tray from the room without contaminating the uniform and taking out all extra dishes, glasses, and medicine glasses.
   c. Scrape the food from the dishes on to the paper.
   d. Pour liquids into a solution of 5 per cent chlorinated lime.
   e. Scrub hands 3 minutes; cover the dishes with water, close the sterilizer and turn on the steam, allowing them to steam 20-30 minutes.
   f. Wrap garbage in the paper on which it is lying and put in the garbage can.

g. Take dishes to the kitchen to be washed.

Transfer of the patients

1. Place a sheet on the cart.
2. Put the patient on the cart.
3. Cover the patient, including the head, with the sheet.
4. Put the linen in the isolated laundry.

Discharge bath

1. Adult:
    a. Nurse puts on a clean gown.
    b. Have the bathroom scrubbed if the patient has used it.
    c. Put a sheet over the patient and lead him to the shower.
    d. Give the patient a bar of soap.
    e. Leave clean towels, wash cloth, and his clean clothing on a chair within reach of the patient.
    f. Place a clean newspaper with a pad on top of it in front of the shower for the patient to step on when he dresses.
    g. Stay within hearing of the patient, and inquire of his condition a couple of times while he is bathing.
    h. Do not allow the patient to go back to the room after bathing.
    i. Take care of the personal belongings of the patient while he is bathing, as scrubbing those that can be scrubbed, putting those to air that need airing, and burning others.
    j. Scrub bed pans with soap and water or sterilize with steam.
    k. Scrub all rubber goods.
    l. Boil all glassware and dishes.
    m. Scrub all furniture in the room and air, taking the bed and mattress out on the open-air porch.
    n. Burn all destructible articles.
    o. Have the porter scrub the walls and wash the floors of the room, corridor, and bathroom.
2. Child:
    a. Wrap him in a sheet and carry him to the bathroom.
3. Bed patient or corpse:
    a. Three clean sheets are put under the patient.
    b. Wash the body with soap and water; as each part of the body is washed, the top sheet is folded back and the bathed part is put on the clean second sheet.
    c. Wrap the body in the second or middle sheet, if it is a corpse.

Miscellaneous instructions

1. Wipe the watch with alcohol.
2. Do not put leather goods in the sterilizer.
3. Air clothing for 3 days in the sunshine.
4. Autoclave mail.

5. Autoclave bills or soak in bichloride of mercury 1-1000 and dry.
6. Sign legal documents by placing the paper on a larger sheet of paper, then covering the document with two more pieces of paper except for the line to be signed.
7. Do not transfer books or magazines from patient to patient.
8. Burn books and magazines upon discharge of patient.

Theory of Aseptic Technique

Minneapolis General Hospital

The theory of aseptic technique is based on the fact that infections are transmitted by actual contact—direct and indirect.

Indirect contact takes place through a contaminated carrier. Air transmission is rare and is therefore not considered of particular importance, except that the doors of rooms occupied by measles patients and smallpox patients are always kept closed. The nurse, however, must be careful not to allow the patient to cough in her face.

Anything that has come directly or indirectly in contact with patients or any infected area is contaminated.

A room or ward occupied by one or more patients representing a separate and distinct infection constitutes a unit. Everything within the unit is considered contaminated.

The aim is to confine each different infection to a separate unit and to prevent the transmission of infection from one unit to another. All areas on the stations not included in units, such as corridors, linen closets, kitchens, etc., are clean.

Gowns supplied for the purpose are worn while treating patients and when cleaning in the unit. Care is taken not to contaminate the inner, clean side of the gown. After the treatment has been done, the hands are washed in the hand solution; the gown is removed and folded so as to cover the inside, and hung on a hook preparatory to being used again. The hands are then scrubbed before treating other patients.

New patients are kept under observation after admission and treated in units of one until two or more reports of nose and throat cultures are received. If these prove satisfactory the patients are moved into wards.

Nurses must remember

1. That the floors in the quarters are contaminated.
2. To wash their hands frequently and always before eating.
3. Not to touch their faces or anything clean when hands are contaminated.
4. Not to allow children to touch their faces.
5. To eat nothing a patient has handled nor to partake of food in a patient's room.

6. To take some out-of-door exercise every day.
7. To sleep with windows open.
8. To take a bath daily.
9. If indisposed to report at once to nurse in charge.
10. To avoid sharing a room with anyone who is ill.
11. To have nose and throat cultures for diphtheria once a week.
12. To always call a person's attention to a breach of technique.
13. To stay away from the stations when off duty.
14. To place their names on their doors in their quarters.
15. To wear a long gown over the ward dress when leaving the floor except on their way to the dressing room in the basement.
16. Sleeves of long gowns must not be rolled. They are to be fastened at the wrist with rubber binders.
17. Contaminated articles must not be placed in waste baskets but burned in the incinerators.
18. Contaminated linen is not to be placed on the floor.
19. Baskets in dressing rooms are to be used for towels only. Nothing contaminated is to be placed in these baskets.
20. Paper sacks are to be used in all patients' rooms.
21. Station telephones are not to be used for outside calls.
22. Nurses have access to the parlors, the classroom, the laundry, and the linen room in the Nurses' Home.
23. Long gowns are not to be worn in the corridors.
24. Students must have nose and throat cultures taken on the day previous to their leaving contagion.

Preparations made for admission of patients

1. The room should contain the fewest possible articles necessary for the care of the patient.
2. Make up foundation of bed only.
3. Equip room with bath tub, wash basin, bed pan, emesis basin, mouth-wash cup, face and bath towels, wash cloth, soap in soap dish, and toilet paper.
4. Thermometer in cup of solution of bichloride of mercury is placed on the shelf.
5. Gown on the hook.
6. Solution of 2 per cent lysol in hand-solution basin.
7. Remove table and chair from side of bed so as not to be in the way when patient is wheeled in.
8. The door of the room is left open.
9. Cart is covered:
   a. Articles necessary:
      (1) Two sheets.
   b. Procedure:
      (1) Fold sheet lengthwise and cover cart, tucking sides under cart pad.

(2) Place spread lengthwise, single thickness, on cart. Fold under. Tuck the sides so that it may cover both sides of the cart, but not touch the wheels.

Admission of patients

1. Patients are admitted in the receiving rooms of the Contagious Department.
2. Patient is carried from the ambulance and placed on the cart.
3. The history is taken, physical examination given, and nose and throat cultures are taken by the interne.
4. Nurse takes the admitting history and makes out the chart.
5. Personal belongings are listed.
6. Patient is transferred to his room. The sides of the spread covering the cart are brought up over the patient covering him completely while he is taken through clean area. At the bedside the side of the sheet covering the patient is pulled down to cover the edge of the cart. The patient is then helped into bed. The blankets and linen in which he is wrapped are used for his bed.

Routine care of newly admitted patients

1. The bed is made up and the patient is made as comfortable as possible.
2. Temperature is taken.
3. Routine orders are carried out according to the disease.
4. Drinking water with glass tube is to be left on stand within easy reach of the patient.
5. Instructions are given to patient:
   a. Patient must not sit up or get out of bed without the doctor's permission.
   b. The floor is contaminated and patient must not pick anything from the floor.

Order of morning work

1. Make a survey of the room to determine what is needed.
2. Get everything ready before becoming contaminated:
   a. Carry into room necessary supplies such as linen, soap, dust cloth, solution of gargle, ice water, ice for ice caps, etc.
   b. Place outside of door, hamper, broom and dust pan, mop and mop pail.
3. Put on mask and long gown.
4. Give patient necessary care:
   a. Bath.
   b. Comb hair.
   c. Cleanse mouth.
   d. See that bed pans and urinals are given at this time to avoid too much handling of patient.

5. Make bed, following instructions on page 19 of this manual (do not allow contaminated linen to fall on the floor. **Place in hamper.**)
6. Sweep the floor. (To avoid raising dust wet the broom before sweeping.)
7. Mop the floor and finish work in room.
8. **Remove gown and hang on hook.**
9. Empty hand-solution basin and refill with water.
10. Push mop pail with mop and carry broom and dust pan to mop closet. Put sweepings in incinerator. **Empty mop pail and scrub handles of broom, mop, mop pail, and dust pan.**
11. Scrub hands for three minutes.
12. Burn contents of incinerator.
13. Wheel hamper to linen chute, tie bag securely so that no contaminated linen is exposed, and drop in chute.
14. Measure out lysol in medicine glass and pour into solution basin in room to make a 2 per cent solution.
15. Scrub glass plate and door knob of patient's room. Care must be taken to avoid having the soapy water run on the wall and door.

Serving of meals

Trays are prepared in the kitchen and carried to the patients' rooms. The nurse's aim must be not to contaminate herself in any way. The tray is placed on the corner of the patient's table or on the edge of his bed and pushed into place by placing fingers against the inner uncontaminated edge of the tray. The door is pushed open with the foot.

Gathering of trays

1. Cover cart with mattress cover allowing it to come down over the edges.
2. Place soup strainer and large basin on cart.
3. Open door of sterilizer.
4. Remove cover of garbage can.
5. Remove trays from the patients' rooms and place on cart. When the nurse has carried the first tray her hands are contaminated. Her aim must be to avoid touching anything except the tray in the patient's room. She opens the door with her elbow. Placing her hand inside of the contaminated tray, she pushes it over the edge of the bed or table so that she may grasp it with the other hand without touching anything but the tray. She then pushes the door open with her foot and places tray on the cart.
6. Scrape and stack the dishes, straining soups, etc. Food remnants are placed in the garbage can in the kitchen and liquids are poured into the hopper in the mop closet.
7. Place the dishes in the sterilizer.

8. Scrub hands for three minutes.
9. Close the door of the sterilizer, turn on the steam, and allow dishes to sterilize for twenty minutes.
10. Replace the cover on the garbage can.
11. Remove ticking from cart, handling from under side.
12. The maid washes the dishes.

Discharge bath and shampoo in tub

When a patient is to be discharged he is given a bath and a shampoo. If the patient is strong enough, the tub in the bathroom may be used. If the patient is unable to be out of bed, a sponge bath is given in his room.

1. Articles needed in bathroom:
   2 bath towels.
   1 face towel.
   1 wash cloth.
   1 cup containing liquid soap.
   1 large pitcher.
   1 hand brush.
   1 sheet.
   1 mattress cover.
   1 bath robe.
2. Articles needed in dressing room:
   1 comb.
   Patient's clothing.
3. General procedure:
   a. Get everything ready in bathroom and dressing room. Water in tub, towels. wash cloth, soap, and pitcher full of warm water on window sill near tub.
   b. Fold mattress cover twice lengthwise. Place on floor leading from bath tub to chair in dressing room.
   c. Cover patient with clean sheet before conducting him from ward to bathroom.
   d. Place sheet on floor, clean side down. Instruct patient to place shirt on the sheet and step into tub. Remove clothing from floor.
   e. Shampoo hair using liquid soap and rinsing with water in pitcher. More water may be had from faucets in tub.
   f. Assist patient in taking his bath. If he is strong enough he may not need assistance. He must then scrub his hands first so that he may be able to manipulate the faucets without contaminating them.
   g. Instruct patient to dry feet carefully before stepping out of tub, to step on mattress cover previously placed for him, to put on clean bath robe, and to walk on mattress cover into dressing room where he may dry his hair and dress in his street clothes.

h. Scrub bath tub (outside as well as inside) and faucets with brown soap and water.

i. Clean and straighten bathroom and dressing room.

Discharge bath in bed

1. Articles needed:

2 sheets.	1 small rubber sheet.
2 blankets.	1 foot tub.
2 face towels.	1 pitcher green soap.
1 wash cloth.	2 large pitchers of water.
3 bath towels.	1 comb.
1 Kelly pad.	1 bed shirt.

2. Procedure:

   a. Move bed to center of room.

   b. Clear table and chair placing table at head of bed and chair near it.

   c. Remove patient's gown and cover him with one of his blankets folded crosswise.

   d. Remove pillows and remaining covers.

   e. Remove contaminated gown and scrub hands.

   f. Cover table and chair with clean sheet and place on these the necessary articles. The foot tub on the chair. Place blanket on top of single thickness of sheet and roll lengthwise. (The cart may be used for this.)

   g. Have patient move to opposite side of bed. Cover bed with roll mentioned above, blanket next patient. Place small rubber sheet under blanket at head of bed, a bath towel on top of this and a Kelly pad in place near the edge of bed. Have patient roll over on Kelly pad and finish covering bed, being careful not to contaminate hands.

   h. Proceed with shampoo as directed on pp. 67-68 in this manual. Hands must be washed in soap and water if accidentally contaminated.

   i. Remove Kelly pad and wrap bath towel around the head.

   j. Proceed to give bath. Wash patient's face, neck, and shoulders, using a generous amount of green soap.

   k. Have patient pull blanket down to waist line. Wash chest.

   l. Wash wrist of arm nearest you. Grasp clean wrist and hold patient's arm away from contaminated bed while washing it. Place clean arm over chest.

   m. Wash opposite arm in same manner and place over chest.

   n. Turn patient on side. Under side of blanket on which patient is lying is clean. Roll this close to patient's back clean side up. Wash back and buttocks.

o. Have patient turn and wash opposite side in same manner. Remove blanket from side of patient so that his lower extremities are resting on it. Put gown on patient.
p. Fold a clean blanket crosswise. Fanfold and place across patient's chest covering him as bath is given.
q. Place small towel over pubis and wash abdomen.
r. Have patient remove cover from extremity nearest and flex his knee. Fold bottom blanket close to foot. Wash leg and thigh.
s. Wash other extremity in same manner.
t. Place foot tub in bed removing blanket. Scrub the feet.
u. Hand soaped wash cloth to patient and instruct him to finish his bath and wash his hands.
v. Dry the hair and comb.

Care of the dead
1. Make all preparations in the same manner as for giving a discharge bath in bed.
2. Moisten the hair with alcohol and dry.
3. Give bath using same procedure as outlined.
4. Get the necessary articles used in the care of the dead and place on clean sheet on table.
5. Proceed as directed on pp. 204-206 of this manual.
6. Take body to morgue in the basement of the contagion building.

How a patient may sign a document without contaminating it
1. Articles needed:
1 chart back.
1 small towel.
4 paper clips.
1 pen.
2. Procedure:
a. Put document on chart back.
b. Cover chart back and document with a towel leaving enough space for signature. Fasten towel with paper clips.
c. Dip pen in ink and hand to patient.
d. After document has been signed, return chart back to chart rack and scrub the penholder.

Care of a laryngeal diphtheria patient
1. Get emergency room (steam room) ready as for an ordinary patient immediately after being told that a patient is coming.
2. Test steam inhaler to see that it is in working order.

3. If steam is ordered, make a croup tent:
  a. Articles needed:
    1 sheet.
    2 safety pins.
  b. General procedure:
    (1) Put up sides of crib.
    (2) Place sheet lengthwise over head of crib and fold end under so as to make the sheet long enough to cover bowl of inhaler and one-third of the length of the crib.
    (3) Fold in corners of sheet and pin with safety pin on each side of bed.
  c. Precautions:
    (1) Do not place crib too close to inhaler.
    (2) Regulate the amount of steam so that patient does not become too warm.
    (3) Never leave patient while steam is being given.
4. Medicated inhalations with steam:
  a. Articles needed:
    1 sheet.
    2 safety pins.
    Medication in hot solution in small kidney basin.
  b. Procedure:
    (1) Make a croup tent.
    (2) Place basin containing hot medicated solution in bowl of inhaler.
    (3) Turn on the steam.
5. Restraining of child for intubation:
  a. Articles needed:
    1 sheet.
    3 safety pins (large).
  b. Procedure:
    (1) Fold sheet lengthwise and place under patient high up at the neck.
    (2) Straighten patient's arms and place at his sides.
    (3) Fold sheet down over right shoulder and wrap end tightly around patient's body.
    (4) Fold sheet over left shoulder and wrap end around patient's body.
    (5) Fasten sheet with safety pins at throat, in front directly in line with elbows, and at the knees.

Care of patient's clothing and personal property
1. An ambulance roll is sent with the ambulance and patient's clothing is left at home:
  a. Ambulance roll:
    2 blankets.

1 bed shirt.
1 sheet.

2. The clothing of patients who are brought to the hospital in private conveyances is sent home if possible; otherwise it is listed in the receiving room in contagion, placed in a bag and left for the orderly to fumigate.

3. No clothing or personal articles are taken from the hospital until properly signed for in the property book.

4. All letters, magazines, toys, books, etc., used by the patient while in the hospital are destroyed after his discharge.

5. Upon death of a patient, personal articles such as rings, watches, mirrors, nail files, etc., in the patient's room are promptly disinfected and left in supervisor's office.

6. Rings and other jewelry must be left in the office where they are properly disinfected and held in the safe. Patients refusing to do this are told that they alone are responsible for their valuables.

7. Money is counted and listed in the presence of the owner. It is then scrubbed with soap and water and before it is placed in the safe it is counted again in the presence of a witness whose signature is put on the envelope with that of the nurse in charge.

Sterilization

1. There are six methods of sterilizing and disinfecting articles used in contagion, namely:
   a. By boiling.
   b. By using steam under pressure in autoclaves.
   c. By scrubbing with soap and water.
   d. By placing articles in antiseptic solutions such as alcohol, lysol, bichloride of mercury, phenol, etc.
   e. By fumigating in air-tight cabinet.
   f. By exposing to fresh air and sunlight.

1. Sterilizing by boiling:
   a. In a dish sterilizer for twenty minutes:
   Dishes, trays, drinking tubes, enamel pitchers, kitchen utensils, white enamel cups, nursing bottles, etc.
   b. In instrument sterilizer:
   (1) White enamel ware, such as kidney basins, soap dishes, dressing bowls, etc.
   (2) Surgical instruments (not sharp).
   (3) Speculi (first to be cleaned with applicators and washed), needles, syringes, etc.
   (4) Rubber tubing, soft rubber catheters, rectal tubes, rubber gloves (for 3 minutes).
   (5) Metal toys.

2. By steam pressure in autoclave:

a. Surgical supplies, rubber gloves.

b. Mattresses, pillows.

c. Letters.

3. By scrubbing with soap and water:

a. Furniture.

b. Large utensils of enamel ware such as bath tubs, bed pans, wash basins, etc.

c. Stethoscope.

d. Rubber sheets, hot water bottles, ice caps, etc.

4. By placing in antiseptic solutions:

a. Sharp instruments as scalpels, scissors, etc. in 95 per cent phenol.

b. Thermometers in phenol.

c. Hard rubber catheters and intubation tubes in 1-1000 bichloride solution for one half hour.

d. Flashlight and otoscope are wiped off very carefully with alcohol. (These must not be boiled, put in solution, or placed in dry sterilizer.)

5. By fumigating in air-tight cabinet:

a. Patient's clothing. (Contaminated articles are not to be placed in paper sacks for fumigation.)

6. By sunlight and fresh air for 24 hours:

a. Leather goods such as restraint straps and cuffs, suitcases, and shoes.

b. Carpet slippers.

c. Light extension cords.

Care of linen

1. Soiled linen is placed in hamper bags on the stations, the dark clothes, such as bath robes, blankets, stockings, etc., being put into dark striped bags made for the purpose.

2. The bags are tied up so as not to expose the contaminated linen while they are dropped into the chute. The orderly then hauls them to the laundry where the linen is sterilized by washing.

How to clean a room after the patient has been discharged

1. Articles needed:

1 mattress cover.

12 safety pins.

1 foot tub.

1 cleaning cloth.

1 hand brush.

1 cake of yellow soap in soap dish.

2. Procedure:

a. Cover cart with mattress cover and place outside of door of room that is to be scrubbed. Also wheel hamper to door (in corridor).

b. Put on the gown (contaminated) which is on the hook.
c. Strip linen off bed and place in hamper bag.
d. Fold mattress with pillows inside and place on the cart. Taking hold of inside of mattress cover, pull ends over mattress.
e. Spread rubber sheet on the bed.
f. Sort all articles in the room.
g. Remove contaminated gown.
h. Place in dish sterilizer all dishes, mouth cups, pitchers, drinking tubes, etc.
i. Place in instrument sterilizer emesis basins, soap dish, etc., being careful to wash them first.
j. Thermometer is washed and placed in phenol basin.
k. Scrub hands.
l. Pin mattress cover over mattress and remove.
m. Put on a clean gown.
n. Scrub top of stand and on it place foot tub and soap dish.
o. Scrub upper side of rubber sheet. Fold and scrub the upper half.
p. Scrub half of bed. Turn rubber sheet over on to the clean area and finish scrubbing it. Dry and hang it over the clean part of the bed.
q. Finish scrubbing the bed.
r. Scrub all furniture and remaining utensils and place on the bed. Finish by scrubbing door knob, window sill, shelf, fixtures, toilet, etc.
s. The windows, walls, and floor are washed by the orderly.
t. The room is made ready for another patient and left to air as long as possible.

The Care of the Isolated Patient
Miller Hospital

The nurse's gown

1. A gown covering the uniform must be worn by the nurse for any work that involves intimate contact with the patient.
2. To put gown on: Remove cuffs and push sleeves to elbow. Hold the gown by neck band and slip one arm in sleeve, then the other. Tie tape at back.
3. To take gown off: Wash hands in liquor cresolis compositus solution 1 per cent, if there is no running water in the room. Slip gown off and crease down center with clean side on inside. If it is to be kept in the room, hang on rod over screen or fold one shoulder within the other and hang on double hook on the screen.

4. If the gown is not worn the nurse must be careful that the uniform does not touch the bed or anything in the room. When caring for one or more patients having the same infection the gown need not be changed between patients. Avoid wearing the gown outside the room. In caring for a patient the nurse should collect everything needed, then put on the gown.

The care of bed linen

1. Place a clean sheet or clothes bag on the floor under the foot of the bed or place on a newspaper on floor in any convenient place.
2. If bag is used: Before contaminating hands, turn back a cuff three or four inches deep. As each piece is taken from the bed place in bag or sheet. When the linen is collected, wash the hands, then close the bag. Tag "Boil," and place by side of clothes hamper.

Care of room

Dust daily, following directions for dusting. Place dust cloth with linen to be boiled. Wash door knobs daily.
Floors: Sprinkle with sweeping compound, sweep floor, collect dust in paper and place in waste pail. The broom should be kept in the room. Before using for another room, scald by running water through hopper.

How to disinfect excreta

1. Use twice as much 5 per cent chloride of lime solution as there is excreta.
2. If feces, break up by using spatula.
3. Expose one hour, or if ordered, longer.
4. Empty pan or urinal and rinse under running water.
5. Keep utensils isolated. When ready to return to general use, boil in sterilizer for fifteen minutes after boiling begins. Clean thoroughly and return to rack.

Secretions

1. Attach a paper bag to bed or bedside table. Use squares of cloth or paper for wiping away secretion, and drop into bag.

Dishes

1. Carry to room on tray.
2. Transfer to second tray or table.
3. Collect in same way, placing upon napkins on tray. Do not contaminate tray.
4. Put refuse food in paper bag to be put into waste pail in service room.
5. Put dishes into boiling water and boil for 15 minutes.

Thermometers
1. Each isolated patient (unless same infection) must have a thermometer.
2. Keep in a bottle of bichloride of mercury 1-1000.
3. Rinse in water before use.
4. After taking the temperature, the nurse must wash her hands before touching chart or temperature book.

Charts
1. Should not be brought to the room. If asked for, clean nurse or physician will hold for reading.

Care of room after discharge or death of isolated patient
1. Care of bed and bedding:
   a. Linen: same as daily care.
   b. Mattress and pillows: must be sent to sterilizer or aired for three days.
   c. Rubber sheets: wash thoroughly with soap and water; air well (one day or longer).
2. Furniture:
   a. Soap and water, air and sunshine are the important factors in disinfection.
   b. Wash bed, bedside table, and all articles of furniture, window ledges, curtain cords, and door knobs.
   c. Air the room one day or longer.

LESSON XIV
THE CARE OF THE DEAD

Aim

1. To have the body straight, clean, and in proper condition for the morgue.

General instructions

1. Note the exact time the patient has ceased to breathe.
2. Lay out the body as soon as the doctor has pronounced the patient dead.
3. Straighten the covers and cover the face with a sheet.
4. See that the body is clean; give special attention to the hair and nails.
5. Do not expose the body unnecessarily.
6. If requested by the hospital administration, a gown and stockings may be put on the body before wrapping in a morgue sheet.
7. Tie bandages in such a way that they will not mark the skin.
8. Do not tell other patients the details of the death and removal of the body.
9. Notify immediately those who are to be told of the death.
10. Treat the body with reverence and always remember that "the body is the temple of the soul." (Kelley.)

Necessary articles

Morgue basket or box containing:
    Morgue sheet.
    Okum pad or cellucotton.
    Comb.
    3 inch bandage.
    Tongue blades.
    Clothes tags.
    Pins.
    Bath and toilet articles.
    Paper bag.
    Toilet paper.
    Ball of twine.
    Safety pins.
    Dressings for a wound, if indicated.

Procedure

1. Close eyes by placing a very thin piece of cotton under the lid.
2. Remove all but two pillows. Leave these to prevent the blood from settling in the head.
3. If patient has false teeth put in the mouth at once.
4. In order to keep the jaw from dropping, prop it with a rolled towel or wide bandage or chin brace.

5. Remove all jewelry and care for it according to the routine of the hospital.
6. Remove all covers except the sheet.
7. Soiled dressings should be replaced with fresh dressings. Remove unattached drainage tubes, artery clamps, etc. Adhesive marks should be removed with benzine.
8. Bathe the body with soap and water. Turn the body on the side, bathe back and at the same time adjust the morgue sheet and pad under the buttocks.
9. Comb the hair and care for the nails.
10. Cross the hands over the chest and tie wrists with a wide bandage in such a way that the wrists will not be marked by the bandage.
11. Fasten a tag to wrists on which is written patient's name, age, registry number, date, and hour of death.
12. Tie knees and ankles together with wide bandage.
13. Fold sheet smoothly around legs, hips, and trunk.
14. Pin down the front and sides, with as few pins as possible, to hold the sheet in place.
15. Bring down over head and pin with safety pin.
16. Fill out second tag the same as first and pin it on the chest.

Record
1. Hour of death.
2. Certified by whom.
3. Anything unusual connected with the death.

Procedure in taking body to morgue
1. Place body on truck and cover with sheet and blanket.
2. See that the elevator is at the floor and that there is no one in the corridor.
3. If an orderly takes the body to the morgue, a nurse must accompany him.
4. Routine reports:
   a. University Hospital:
      (1) Triplicate death notices are made out and one is sent to the school of nursing office, one goes with the body, and one to the superintendent of the hospital.
      (2) Put name, hour of death, and service on census slip.
      (3) Remove card from diet chart and cross off name on defecation chart.
   b. Miller Hospital:
      (1) Same as number 2 and 3 under University Hospital.
      (2) Three notification slips are made out by head nurse; one sent to the superintendent of the hospital, one to the superintendent of nurses, and one to the main office.
      (3) See that the pathologist is notified.

(4) Cross off name on daily report sheet.
(5) White stockings and gown are put on, and chin brace must be used.
(6) A charge slip is made out for gown, large pad, sheet, and stockings. Patient may use own if available.

c. N. P. B. A. Hospital.
(1) Entire responsibility of reports taken care of by staff and internes.
(2) Clothing must be checked and wrapped and go with the body to the morgue.
(3) All valuables are listed and taken to the business office.
(4) Morgue key is obtained from business office.

d. Minneapolis General Hospital:
(1) Take patient's name from census board.
(2) Place the body in a compartment in the morgue and insert the name slip in the holder in the door.
(3) Fill out the morgue sheet with patient's name, date, and hour put in morgue.
(4) Triplicate death notices are sent out, two to information desk and one to school of nursing office.

Care of patient's belongings

1. All rings, ear rings, bracelets, beads, and emblems of sacred or religious meaning should be removed, listed, and placed in a package with other articles of value such as money, receipts, eyeglasses, letters, keys, etc. At top of list write patient's name and register number and care for package according to the routine of the hospital.
2. All clothing and other personal property should be checked, wrapped neatly in a bundle, properly tagged, and taken to the property room (General Hospital) or morgue.
3. Any person removing valuables or personal belongs of deceased from the hospital, must sign a statement to that effect.

DUTIES OF THE NIGHT NURSE
Day and Night Reports
University Hospital

1. Fill in all headings at top of sheet.
2. If it is the day report, draw a line through A. M. If it is the night report, vice versa.
3. List all patients' names about whom it is necessary to report in the space provided.
4. On the other side of the line, directly opposite the patient's name, write the ward letter, diagnosis, and condition.
5. The report must be printed neatly and properly signed.
6. A carbon copy is made, the carbon being kept in the station and the original taken to the school office before 6:30 P.M.

Duties of the 11 O'clock Nurse
University Hospital

1. Report on duty at 6:30 P. M.
2. Read doctor's orders. Carry out "stat" orders or any others due.
3. Read nurse's evening report.
4. Take evening temperatures and chart.
5. Give nourishment per diet list.
6. Read med. cards: red, green, and white.
7. Pour medicine according to cards and doctor's orders.
8. See that medicine is taken by patient.
9. Check and chart.
10. Dismiss visitors promptly at 8 P. M.
11. Put out corridor ceiling lights.
12. Fill ice bags and hot water bags.
13. See that every bed patient has fresh water.
14. If possible have every patient use a bed pan.
15. Remove flowers to corridor.
16. Leave wards in perfect order.
17. Put ward lights out at 8:45.
18. Wash nourishment dishes and leave diet kitchen in order.
19. See that service rooms are clean and in order.
20. Do not give p. r. n. orders without permission from night supervisor.
21. Report to night nurse.
22. Report to night supervisor in office.

Duties of the Night Nurse
University Hospital

1. Report to night supervisor in main office at 10:30 P. M. Receive reports of 11:00 nurse.

Read night orders in night order book and doctor's order book.
Carry out any "stat" orders.

2. Make rounds to ascertain condition of patients. See new patients and find out immediate needs before beginning routine work of night.

3. From doctor's order book and medication and treatment cards make a list of medications and treatments with time to be given during the night.
This is for your own use; refer to it often.
Carry out all orders promptly and chart and check in doctor's order book immediately *after* order has been carried out.

4. Make rounds every hour during the night. Go to the bedside of every patient, and note whether patient is asleep or awake. Watch condition of all patients carefully at all times during night, special observation being made of new patients and those who are seriously ill.

5. Report at once to the night supervisor any alarming symptoms or sudden change in a patient's condition.

6. From specimen chart and doctor's order book make a list of the number and kind of specimen bottles needed for the morning use. Give the night orderly this requisition at 11:00 P. M. Fill out laboratory request blanks as soon as time permits. Rule temperature books leaving sufficient space for q. 4 h. temperatures. When a temperature is to be taken by rectum or axilla, make this notation both in book and on chart.

7. Rule charts as near midnight as possible.
Keep charts of seriously ill patients nearest at hand.

8. Rule doctor's book in red ink promptly at 12:00 (important), e. g., doctor's order 5-8-22.

9. Do not give an s. o. s. order for medication or treatment without the approval of the night supervisor.

10. Give good nursing care before reporting a patient as wakeful. A warm alcohol rub, a hot water bottle, or glass of hot milk (if diet does not contraindicate) is often very effective.

11. Give special attention to ventilation. Use screens to protect patients from drafts or necessary light. Always keep patients well covered using extra blankets when needed. This is very important in the care of children.

12. Write night report after 4:00 A. M. Outline may be made earlier. Important medications and treatments given patient during night should be mentioned, also elevated temperatures. Make report worthy of going on file and do not omit signature.

13. Routine A. M. charting of patients' conditions should be done after 4:00 A. M.
With seriously ill patients, some notation concerning condition should be made at least q. 2. h.

14. Give routine A. M. care after 5:00 A. M. Bed pans, wash basins, and mouth wash should be given to all bed patients. Assist the very sick patients and see that patients permitted to go to the bathroom have completed their toilet by 6:45 A. M. In the male wards the orderly helps with the morning care, but the nurse is held responsible for this supervision and she should assist with the care of the seriously ill.

15. Complete the 24 hour specimens as near 6:00 A. M. as possible. Morning specimens to be ready as soon after 6:00 A. M. as possible and sent to the laboratory not later than 7:00 A. M. Explain to new patients the importance of obtaining accurate 24 hour specimens and try to gain their cooperation. Total intakes and outputs and chart at 6:00 A. M., note and report any apparent inconsistency.
Care should be taken to collect urine from all diabetic patients to complete the twenty-four hour specimen.

16. Try to plan your work well, always allowing sufficient time for emergencies that will often delay your routine.

17. Wards, diet kitchens, service rooms, linen rooms, and cupboards are to be left in order.

18. Clean corridor desks and bowls during night.

19. Be prepared to give verbal report to day nurses promptly at 7:00 A. M.

20. Send A. M. specimen of urine on all new patients the morning after admission.

Order of Night and Day Reports
N. P. B. A. Hospital

Census

Admissions

1. Name.
2. Private or N. P. patient.
3. Room.
4. Time.
5. Diagnosis.
6. Condition.

Discharge

1. Name.
2. Private or N. P. patient.
3. Room.
4. Time.

Death
1. Name.
2. Private or N. P.
3. Room.
4. Time and doctor's name.

Transfers
1. Name.
2. Private or N. P.
3. Room number.
4. Time.

Births
1. Name.
2. Sex.
3. Time.

Cathartic list

Sedative list

Urinalysis list

List of patients according to wards and room numbers
1. Beginning at the central desk and going down the corridor in order and give a definite and concise record of the patient's condition.
2. Day report:
   a. Note all medications, treatments, and orders for patients between 7:00 A. M. and 7:00 P. M., making such notations as taking a patient off diet or putting him on diet.
3. Night report:
   a. Record all work done for patient between 7:00 P. M. and 7:00 A. M., making all statements about operation orders, x-rays, Ewald meals, Hawdek meals, etc.

General instructions
a. Print the report.
b. Do not use expressions as: "fine night," "feels O. K.," "slept well," etc.
c. Do not use incorrect abbreviations.
d. Keep charts and order book neat; both are kept as evidence.
e. Sign the report.

Duties of the Night Nurse

N. P. B. A. Hospital

1. Report to the dining room at 10:30 for supper.
2. Receive relief nurse's report at 11:00 P. M.

3. Read doctor's order book and report book.
4. Carry out any "stat" orders.
5. Make a list of orders and time they are to be carried out from the doctor's order book, report book, and the medication and treatment cards.
6. Carry out all orders promptly, chart, and check in the doctor's order book immediately after the order has been carried out.
7. Make complete rounds q. 2 h. during the night; go to the bedside of every patient and note whether the patient is asleep or awake. Seriously ill patients receive constant attention, or attention about every 15 minutes.
8. Report at once to the night supervisor any alarming or sudden change in a patient's condition.
9. Rule charts as near midnight as possible; keep charts of seriously ill patients nearest at hand.
10. Rule doctor's order book in red ink promptly at midnight as: "Doctor's orders 8-22-28."
11. Do not give a p. r. n. order for a medication or treatment without the approval of the night supervisor.
12. Give good nursing care such as a warm alcohol rub, hot water bottle to the feet, or a glass of hot milk if not contraindicated by the diet, before reporting a patient as wakeful.
13. Give special attention to ventilation; use screens to protect patients from drafts or necessary light. Always keep patients well covered, using extra blankets when needed. (This is very important when caring for children.)
14. Be sure that the heading of the chart is carried over correctly each night, changing the room number if the patient has been transferred, and the doctor's name if the service has been changed.
15. Write the night report after 4:00 A. M., the outline may be made earlier. All important medications, treatments, elevated temperatures, or changed conditions from 7:00 P. M. to 7:00 A. M. are recorded.
16. Do all routine A. M. charting after 4:00 A. M. except for seriously ill patients; that is done last. Charting concerning sick patients is done at least q. 2 h. during the night.
17. Give preoperative enema at 5:30 A. M.
18. Pass bed pans, first, after 6:00 A. M.; then the mouth wash and wash basins. Assist the very sick patients and see that all the up patients complete their toilets by 6:45 A. M.
19. Total intakes and outputs, including proctoclysis, at 6:00 A. M., and chart.
20. Complete 24 hour specimens as near 6:00 A. M. as possible. Obtain, check, and chart all specimens on those requested, preoperative, two days postoperative, new patients. (If some

are not obtained, report it at morning circle, when all students gather around desk with the head nurse for A. M. report.

21. Pass fresh drinking water before 7:00 A. M.
22. Have the night report written by 6:30 for the night supervisor to see.
23. Leave wards, room, diet kitchens, service room, cupboards, and linen cupboards in order before 7:00 A. M. Take basins out of sterilizer.
24. Clean desks before 7:00 A. M.
25. Check up on routine orders as salicylates, pre- and postoperative cases like hemorrhoidectomies, gynecological cases, and x-ray.
26. Plan the work so that there will be sufficient time for emergencies.

Duties of Relief and Night Nurses
(7:00-11:00 p. m. and 11:00-7:00 a. m., Respectively)
Minneapolis General Hospital

Routine duties

1. On duty at 7:00 P. M.
2. Day report of condition of patients, treatment during day, and treatment ordered for night, by head nurse.
3. Be sure all orders are understood before head nurse leaves the station.
4. Locate new patients and see all serious patients and operatives.
5. Make a list in temperature book and take T. P. R. of:
   a. All patients with temperature of 100° or over.
   b. All seriously ill patients.
   c. All patients having subnormal temperature.
6. Give q-4-h, b. i. d., and q. i. d. medicines at 8:00 P. M., cathartics are also to be given at night, and other medications as ordered.
7. Sleep-producing medicines:
   a. Prior to fulfilling these orders, have the patient ready for sleep: bed comfortable, treatment given, temperature taken, visitors excluded, ventilation as perfect as possible. After the medicine is given, add the finishing touches, give a drink of water, adjust the light. Keep room quiet.
8. Give all treatments when ordered.
9. See that bed pans are passed to all patients and attend to all their wants.
10. See that patients have extra blankets for night and that there is good ventilation in wards.
11. Make all seriously ill patients as comfortable as possible. Remember that doing this at bedtime insures a better night for the patient and less disturbance in the ward later on.
12. See that all lights are out in wards at 9:00 P. M.

13. After patients are settled, chart temperatures, medicine, and condition of patients before midnight.
14. Supper served from 11-12. Never leave station alone. On station where there is only one nurse the night supervisor arranges for relief.
15. After midnight, draw midnight line. All night charting to be done in red ink. Put on new chart sheets if necessary and draw temperature and pulse line to edge of each sheet.
16. Complete daily census slip (Form 132). Make rounds and count patients to make sure it is correct. Take to information desk at midnight.
17. Fill out doctor's report slips putting all patients' names of same service on one slip (Form 287).
18. Take T. P. R. of all patients at midnight, according to Rule 4. If patient is sleeping do not awaken to take temperature unless ordered.
19. A. M. lunch served on Station A. Each nurse must wash her own dishes and leave kitchen in good order.
20. Take 4:00 A. M. temperatures as above.
21. Begin A. M. work at 5:00 A. M. Give all A. M. treatments and pass bed pans to bed patients. Collect and label all specimens to be sent to laboratory. These are taken to laboratory by orderly.
22. After bed pans and urinals are used, collect all and put to soak, adding 4 cups floor powder to one tub water.
23. Pass basins and mouth wash to all bed patients. Wash the hands and faces of all helpless and very sick patients. Be sure that every patient on the station has had this care.
24. Pass mouth wash to up patients and see that they make their morning toilets.
25. Finish charting, write the night report in report book, and send a copy to School of Nursing office.

Night Report

Station D   April 20th, 1922.
Census
No. admitted
No. discharged
No. transferred
No. died
Ward I
a. Make report concise and legible, using correct spelling and stating only important facts about patients.
b. Write report in consecutive order, reporting on all patients in Ward I, and then Ward II, etc.
c. Report on all seriously ill patients. Write first and last name T. P. R., at 8:00 P. M. and A. M., important treatments

and medications during night, condition of patient, and kind and amount of sleep. Unusual symptoms.
d. Report anything unusual that happens on ward.
26. Pass saline cathartics at 6:00 A. M. unless otherwise ordered. Pass all A. C. medicines between 6:00 and 7:00 A. M.
27. General tidying of service rooms, bathrooms, and wards. See that soiled linen is sent down chute. Blankets are put under spreads. Bed covers straightened, and beds lined up in straight rows, shades taken off lights. See that kitchen is in good order.
28. Clean head nurse's desk and other desks; put on clean blotter pads, wash pens, and refill inkwells.
29. Read night report to head nurse at 7:00 A. M.

Routine for Night Nurses

Miller Hospital

1. *Always* carry the master key and *keep cupboards locked.*
2. Check narcotics at 11:00 P. M. and 7:00 A. M.
3. Call night supervisor:
   a. Whenever in doubt.
   b. For permission to give narcotics.
   c. For carrying out of p. r. n. orders.
   d. Report any change in a patient's condition immediately.
4. Read doctor's order book *carefully* and check orders when carried out, stating time.
5. Rule doctor's order book at midnight.
6. Start morning report not earlier than 4:00 A. M.
7. Do not call internes without notifying night supervisor, unless called by a doctor.
8. When filling sterilizers do not leave, if called away, without turning the water off.
9. Night supervisor expects a report of patients when making rounds.
10. Turn off dripping taps.
11. Have a report from special nurses by 6:30 A. M.
12. Laboratory request for patients going to be surgical on that day should be marked "for operation" in red ink.

APPENDIX B
OPERATIVE ROUTINE
Preoperative Routine
University Hospital

Aim

1. To make the patient, especially at the site of the operation, as clean as possible, and thus remove one source of infection of the wound.
2. To empty the stomach, intestines, and bladder so that:
   a. The intestines and bladder will not discharge their contents when the sphincter muscles are relaxed under the influence of the anesthetic.
   b. An incision will not be made accidently in any of these organs as sometimes happens in an abdominal operation when they are distended.
   c. The entrance of solid substance into the trachea will be prevented; this is a very probable occurence if there is solid food in the stomach.
   d. The intense nausea and auto-intoxication that are apt to follow general anesthesia if there is much food in the intestine or stomach will be prevented.
3. To see that the patient has as much rest as possible before operation to insure a good recovery.

General preparation

1. Bath and shampoo 12-24 hours before.
2. Cathartic afternoon before per doctor's orders.
3. Light diet at supper unless contraindicated or a case where diet is specified.
4. No water after midnight.
5. S. s. colon flush A. M. of operation. Repeat until clear.
6. No breakfast.

Local preparation

1. Necessary articles (on tray) :
   Basin of sterile water.
   Sterile green soap.
   Sterile cotton balls.
   Applicators with cotton.
   Safety razor with blades.
   Paper bag.
   Paper square (tissue).
   2 rubber protectors.
   2 towels—1 bed-pan cover in a perineal case.
   Alcohol.
   Benzene.
   Kidney basin.

2. Method:
   a. Wash hands.
   b. If other than rectal or perineal case, place towels over rubber and place on either side of area to be shaved.
   c. Soap area well and shave per "Directions for Area to be Prepared for Various Operations."
   d. After shaving wash area well with soap and water.
   e. If necessary clean umbilicus with alcohol. Be sure it is clean before leaving patient.
3. After-care of articles:
   a. Take razor apart and very carefully put in kidney basin filled with ½ per cent liquor cresolis compositus solution. Let stand for 15 minutes, then wash with soap and water, rinse, and dry thoroughly. Be careful not to let blade knock against any hard surface. Keep used blades in one compartment in box, and new in other compartment.
   b. Boil other basins used, and replace clean on tray.
   c. Leave tray clean and with all necessary articles on it.

Final preparation
   1. Entirely cover the hair with a triangular bandage; for female patient, comb hair in two braids and cover completely, using no safety pins.
   2. Remove false teeth or removable bridge. Keep in cup of boric acid solution in locked closet until such time as the patient may need them.
   3. Thoroughly cleanse mouth.
   4. Remove all jewelry. At the head nurse's discretion a ring may be worn. (This should be tied with a tape to the wrist.)
   5. Have patient empty bladder. Measure and record time and amount of urine voided. Notify head nurse if patient is unable to void and she will notify the physician. Do not catheterize without an order.
   6. If the operation is abdominal only, or upon the upper body, put on ether stockings and pin blanket neatly about the legs and over the feet.
   7. Ether stockings are put on all cases.
   8. If a hypodermic of morphine has been ordered preliminary to the anesthetic, this should be given after any preparation that will occasion any disturbance of the patient has been done; it is usually given ½ hour before the patient goes to the operating room.

Postoperative Routine
University Hospital

Aim
   1. To prevent the occurrence of complications.
   2. To counteract the effect of the operation.

Procedure

1. Make up ether bed.
2. Remove hot water bags from bed and turn back covers.
3. Put patient in bed.
4. Put on dry gown if necessary.
5. Cover patient well, especially around shoulders.
6. If patient is covered with perspiration, dry with towel; a bath towel is preferable.
7. Turn the head to one side and wash out the mouth after each emesis.
8. Hold up jaw with fingers underneath if the patient is not breathing well.
9. Record the pulse every 15 minutes.
10. Note the condition of skin.
11. Note when patient is conscious and chart.
12. Do not restrain the patient too much.
13. Allow plenty of fresh air without causing a draught.
14. Have the room shaded.
15. Straighten up the room.
16. Tuck in covers at foot of bed and have bed as neat as possible.
17. *Do not leave patient until he is conscious.*
18. Measure all urine voided for at least 3 days after operation and longer if patient is not voiding the right amount.

Watch for the following conditions

a. Shock:
   (1) Nervous system depressed.
   (2) Muscular tissue of the heart, blood vessels, and other viscera is relaxed.
   (3) Blood collects in the larger blood vessels and the circulation in the smaller vessels is very poor.
   (4) Body becomes cold.
   (5) Notify head nurse. Treatment: apply external heat, elevate foot of bed, give stimulants.
b. Hemorrhage.
c. Retention of urine.
d. Dilated stomach:
   (1) An accumulation of gas in intestines and then into stomach is due to lack of tone and the stomach fails to contract as it should.
   (2) Treatment: lavage, enemata, medication.
e. Acidosis
   (1) Irritation of mucous membranes of lungs caused by ether.
   (2) Diminished oxidation.
   (3) Defective metabolism.
   (4) Accumulation of toxins.
f. Infection.
g. Pneumonia.

    h. Thrombus.
    i. Peritonitis.

To make patient comfortable

1. To relieve thirst, dip gauze in ice water and rinse out the mouth.
2. Wipe lips with lemon juice, glycerine, or albolene.
3. Wash out the mouth after each emesis.
4. Give water when ordered.
5. Sponge the face with cool water and wash the hands.
6. After emesis have linen clean.
7. Place a small pillow under small of back to prevent cramping.
8. Give proctoclysis for thirst.
9. Place a rolled pillow under knees.
10. Change position.
11. Place cold compresses on forehead or on neck (for nausea).
12. Sponge back and rub with alcohol at night.
13. Keep foundation bed free from wrinkles.
14. Give food with discretion; pay particular attention to preferences and dislikes of patient.

Gastrostomy

1. Articles necessary:
   Graduated glass or pitcher.
   Small funnel with 12 inches of tubing.
   Glass connecting tube to connect with catheter.
   Solution as ordered.
2. Method:
   a. Expel air from tubing by pouring a small amount of the fluid into the tubing.
   b. Unclamp end of catheter, insert end of connecting tube, and let the fluid in very slowly.
   c. Never allow the funnel to become empty.
   d. Be careful of catheter.

Eye Operations

General preparation

1. Same as for other operations except liquids only are usually given for supper.

Local preparation

1. Lid operation:
   a. Wash field with soap and water, then alcohol, and follow with 1-1000 bichloride solution.
   b. Cover field with sterile dressing.
2. Eyeball operation:
   a. Same procedure as shown above, only no dressing at night. Pay particular attention to cleansing eyebrows. Do not clip eyelashes without order, enucleation excepted.

Postoperative care
1. Usual care of bed patients.
2. Patient to remain quiet for the first 24 hours, then he may be turned carefully on either side.
3. Put mask on patient at night to protect eyes while he sleeps.
Note: Cataract cases
  1. Diet:
    a. Liquids first day.
    b. Semisolid diet second day and until patient sits up, then light or general diet.
  2. Give no cathartic until fifth day following operation.

Throat Operations

General preparation
1. Same as for other operations. Varies some according to patient.

Postoperative care
1. No water for 2 hours after operation; may have chipped ice.
2. Watch for bleeding.
3. Ice bag to neck p. r. n.
4. Mouth wash p. r. n. 24 hours after operation.
5. Liquid or semisolid diet, whichever the patient wishes.

Preparation of Gynecology Cases

University Hospital

General preparation
1. Same as for other operations.
2. Vaginal douche A. M. and P. M.

Local preparation
1. Shaving of abdomen.
2. Shaving of pelvic floor.
3. Just before the patient is taken to the operating room, wash the vulva, lower abdomen, inner surface of thighs, and buttocks with liquid soap. Apply sterile perineal pad and T binder.
4. Omit blanket.
5. All rectal and genito-urinary cases are prepared the same way.

Directions for Area to Be Prepared for Various Operations

University Hospital

Abdominal operation
1. Shave from breasts to low on pubes and 4-5 inches on either side of median line.
2. Scrub from breast to pubes and to bed line on either side.

Stomach (same as for abdominal operation)
1. Shave from breasts to below umbilicus and 4-5 inches on either side of median line.
2. Scrub from breast to pubes and to bed line on either side.

Kidney
1. Shave and scrub from sternum to the spine on the affected side and from axilla to the hip.

Breast
1. Shave axilla, chest on affected side to umbilicus, and upper arm to elbow.
2. Scrub from hair line and ear to waist line, from nipple on opposite side to behind shoulder on the affected side, including upper arm.

Neck
1. Shave from hair line to nipple, axilla, and shoulder on affected side.
2. Scrub from hair line to below nipple, axilla, shoulder, and upper arm.

Scalp
1. Order usually given by surgeon as to extent of surface to be prepared.
2. It is an offense to shave larger areas than necessary. Therefore, to protect the hospital and to insure safe preparation of the patient, the order must be written if there are no written routine orders for the ward.

Leg or arm
1. Shave and prepare well above and below the affected part.

Special operation: eye, ear, nose, throat, skin graft, etc.
1. Preparation varies with condition and operation.
2. Routine orders usually written for use of ward. If not, order must be written for each patient.

Vaginal and rectal operations
1. Place the patient in the dorsal position. Shave the pubes and skin surrounding the vulva and anus. Scrub the lower abdomen, upper one-third of thigh, and inner surfaces of thighs and buttocks.
2. Male patients should be prepared by operating room or floor orderly.

Vein-stripping operation
1. Shave pubes and leg to be operated on.

Routine for General Anesthesia
N. P. B. A. Hospital

1. At 4 P. M., the charge nurse reports to the main office for the list of operations for the following day. These names and orders are transferred to the doctor's order book.
2. Take the patient off diet.
3. Preoperative tray ordered from the special diet kitchen.
4. Field of operation is prepared before 7 A. M.
   a. Bone cases: Field of operation is to be painted with mercurochrome 2 per cent morning of operation and sterile towel applied, fastened with a bandage.
5. S. s. enema at 6 A. M. day of operation.
6. Preoperative hypodermic ½ hour before going to surgery. Give morphine sulphate gr. 1/6 and atropine sulphate gr. 1/150 unless otherwise ordered.
7. Remove false teeth and put into a cup of mouth wash.
8. Remove all jewelry, put it in an envelope, and give to the supervisor. The wedding ring may be tied on with a bandage.
9. The patient wears a short gown, bath robe, shoes, and stockings to the operating room.
10. Patient voids before going to the operating room.
11. Enteroclysis of 2000 cc. tap water is prepared to be given to the patient on return from the operating room except thyroidectomies, hemorrhoidectomies, anal fistulas, and anyone who is conscious.

Routine orders

1. Hemorrhoid cases:
   a. Saline enema at 7 P. M. night before operation and 6 A. M. morning of operation.
   b. Mineral oil, ounces 1, b. i. d. beginning the morning following the operation.
   c. Soft diet morning following the operation.
   d. Oleum ricini, ounces 1, at 6 A. M. on the fifth day following operation.
   e. Up on the fifth day and full diet. Discontinue mineral oil b. i. d. and give it, ounces, 1, once a day.
2. Thyroidectomies
   a. Remain in bed the morning of operation.
   b. Up in Fowler's position on return from the operating room.
   c. Wound dressed at 8:30 P. M. on day of operation.
3. Gastroenterostomies, cholecystectomies, hysterectomies, and drainage cases:
   a. Up in Fowler's position when conscious.
   b. Gastroenterostomies receive no water by mouth until doctor orders it.

4. Tonsillectomies:
  a. General:
    (1) All children 4 years old or over to have atropine sulphate, gr. 1/200, by hypodermic 30 minutes before operation.
    (2) Wrap children under 6 years of age in a bath blanket.
    (3) On return from surgery, children lie in a prone position.
  b. Local:
    (1) All adults to have atropine sulphate, gr. 1/150, by hypodermic ½ hour before going to the operating room.
    (2) Patients wear long gowns, bath robe, shoes, and stockings. Women wear a triangular bandage over their heads.
5. Teeth extraction (general, Dr. Barnett):
  a. Morphine sulphate, gr. ¼, and atropine sulphate, gr. 1/150, by hypodermic ½ hour before going to surgery.
  b. Instruct the patient not to rinse his mouth the first day of operation.
6. Nasal cases (Dr. Nordin):
  a. Give a breakfast of 2 pieces of toast with coffee on the morning of the operation.
  b. Give soda barbital, gr. VII ss., 45 minutes before the operation.
  c. Soft diet night of operation.
  d. After the splints are removed, nasal pill is to be used t. i. d.
  e. Phenacetin, gr. V, if necessary for headache on day of operation only.
  f. Fibrogen 2 cc. intramuscularly for considerable bleeding.
  g. Give nasal oil, oz. 2, upon discharge from hospital.
7. Eye cases (Dr. Nelson):
  a. Dilatation of pupils:
    (1) One drop of homatropine in each eye q. 15 minutes for 3 doses.
8. Abdominal cases:
  a. Before going to the surgery, wash the abdomen with ether and paint with a 2 per cent mercurochrome solution.
9. Bone cases:
  a. Before going to the surgery, wash the area with ether, paint with a 2 per cent mercurochrome solution, and bandage with a sterile towel fastened with a bandage. (Use no pins or safety pins.)
  b. A rubber pillow case on a pillow is to accompany the patient to the surgery.
10. Gynecological cases:
  a. A 2 per cent boric acid douche is to be given on the morning of the operation.

Directions for Area to Be Prepared for Various Operations

N. P. B. A. Hospital

Abdominal operation
1. Shave from breasts to low on pubes and to bed line on either side of patient.
2. Scrub from breast to pubes and to bed line on either side.

Stomach
1. Shave from breasts to below umbilicus and to bed line on either side of patient.
2. Scrub from breast to pubes and to bed line on either side.

Kidney
1. Shave and scrub from sternum to the spine and from axilla to the hip on the affected side.

Breast
1. Shave axilla, chest on affected side, and upper arm.
2. Scrub from hair line and ear to waist line, from nipple on opposite side to behind shoulder on the affected side, including upper arm.

Neck
1. Shave from hair line to nipple, axilla, and shoulder on affected side.
2. Scrub from hair line to below nipple, axilla, shoulder, and upper arm.

Scalp
1. Order usually given by surgeon as to extent of surface to be prepared.
2. It is an offence to shave larger area than necessary. Therefore, to protect the hospital and to insure safe preparation of the patient, the order must be written if there are no written routine orders for the ward.

Leg or arm
1. Shave and prepare well above and below the affected part.

Special operations: eye, ear, nose, throat, skin graft, etc.
1. Preparation varies with condition and operation.
2. Routine orders usually written for use of ward. If not, order must be written for each patient.

Vaginal and rectal operation
1. Place the patient in the dorsal position.
2. Shave the pubes and skin surrounding the vulva and anus.
3. Scrub the lower abdomen, upper third of thigh, and inner surfaces of thighs and buttocks.

4. Male patients should be prepared by operating room or floor orderly.
5. When radium is to be inserted into the cervix or uterus, clip the hair over the perineum; do not shave.
6. For any rectal case, clip the hair over the perineum and shave an area 3 to 4 inches in diameter around the anus.

General Preparation of Patient for Operation

Minneapolis General Hospital

General preparation
1. Tub bath night before if possible.
2. Sponge bath day before:
   a. Inspect finger and toe nails and umbilicus.
3. Carry out doctor's orders:
   a. Cathartic night before.
   b. Enema early in A. M.
   c. Light supper, liquids until midnight, *no breakfast.*
   d. Hypodermic as ordered, to be charted when given.

Local preparation
1. Shaving done by dressing room nurses or orderly, usually night before.

Final preparation (nurse in ward responsible)
1. Teeth cleaned.
2. Binder inspected.
3. Inspect finger and toe nails.
4. Braid and comb hair tightly and pin up in towel as for pediculosis cap.
5. Remove false teeth, place in water, and put in safe place.
6. Remove jewelry and give to head nurse.
7. Put on clean gown and surgical stockings.
8. Have patient void within ½ hour of going to operating room. If patient is unable to void report to head nurse. *This is important.*
9. See that chart is ready. Chart hour patient goes to operating room.
10. Do not forget the human element in the preparation. Talk to patient and assure him about operation. Put yourself in patient's place.

Local Preparation for Operation

Minneapolis General Hospital

Aim
1. To make the site of operation as clean as possible, thus removing one source of infection of the wound.

Articles needed

Razor.
Toilet paper.
Emesis basin.
Compresses.
Green soap.

General instructions

1. Male patients are to be shaved by orderly.
2. Because the iodine preparation used in the operating room will not penetrate if water has been used on the surface within 12 hours, patient must be prepared the day before operation. *Emergency cases must be shaved dry.*
3. Avoid cutting skin.
4. It is important to scrub surface thoroughly with soap and hot water in order to cleanse the numerous small ducts in the skin and remove the fatty excretion and dried epithelium from the surface.
5. Be sure that the umbilical area is scrupulously clean.
6. Areas to be prepared for different operations:
   a. Abdominal:
   Shave from breasts over pubes and five inches on either side of median line. Scrub from breasts to pubes and to bed line on either side.
   b. Stomach:
   Shave from breasts to below umbilicus and five inches on either side of median line. Scrub from breasts to pubes and to bed line on either side.
   c. Kidney:
   Shave and scrub from sternum to the spine on the affected side and from axilla to hip.
   d. Breast:
   Shave axilla, chest on affected side, and upper arm. Scrub from hair line and ear to waist line, from nipple on opposite side to behind shoulder on the affected side, including upper arm.
   e. Neck:
   Shave from hair line to nipple, axilla, and shoulder on affected side. Scrub from hair line to below nipple, axilla, shoulder, and upper arm.
   f. Scalp:
   Order given by surgeon as to extent of surface to be prepared. To protect hospital definite order must be written.
   g. Leg or arm:
   Shave and prepare well above and below the affected part.
   h. Vaginal and rectal operation:
   Place patient in the dorsal position. Shave the pubes and

skin surrounding the vulva and anus. Scrub the lower abdomen, upper third of thigh, and inner surfaces of thighs and buttocks. Male patients are prepared by orderly.

i. Special operation (eye, ear, nose, and throat):
Preparation varies with condition and operation. Order written for each patient.

Procedure

1. Ordinary washing of hands.
2. Saturate compress with soap and water and lather surface.
3. Shave, using toilet paper to remove hair.
4. Saturate compress with soap and water, scrub area thoroughly. Repeat this several times.
5. Saturate compress with water, wash area. Repeat several times.

Postoperative Care of Patients

Minneapolis General Hospital

Aim

1. To care for patient during recovery from anesthesia so as:
   a. To lessen shock.
   b. To observe promptly any change.
   c. To prevent patient from injuring himself.

General instructions

1. Never leave an unconscious patient alone.

Procedure

1. Immediate care:
   a. Turn down bed and remove jugs or hot water bottles.
   b. Assist in lifting patient from stretcher to bed.
   c. Tuck blankets closely about patient.
   d. Turn patient's head on side; adjust towel under chin.
   e. Take pulse and respirations q-10 minutes, until patient is conscious, longer if he is not in good condition.
   f. Take T. P. R. q-4-h for 48 hours after operation.
   g. Observe:
      (1) General condition (unconscious, semiconscious, conscious).
      (2) Symptoms (skin: color; quality of pulse and respiration; vomitus; restlessness; stain on dressings, etc.).
2. Later care:
   a. Water given as ordered (lips may be moistened or patient may rinse mouth with water without order).
   b. Six to eight hours after return from operating room, remove extra blanket, unfasten binder, and give alcohol rub. Have patient void, and measure urine. Make comfortable with pillows, pads, etc. Patient may be turned on side if com-

fortable in that position. Pillow may be placed under head if not nauseated.
c. If proctoclysis has been given, observe amount retained and chart.
3. Charting:
a. Transfer notes and pulse and respiration from scratch pads to chart.

Preparation of Patients for Operation

Miller Hospital

General external preparation (entire body must be scrupulously clean)
1. Cleansing tub bath before putting into clean bed if patient is able to take tub bath. If not able to take tub bath, patient must have thorough cleansing bed bath.
2. If necessary and there is time, wash patient's hair. Inspect for vermin in hair.
3. Trim and clean patient's finger and toe nails.
4. Pay special attention to umbilicus. This is most important.
5. Send specimen of urine to laboratory (get as soon as possible after admission). Mark in red ink: "Specimen," "For operation," with date and hour of operation.

Local preparation of area of operation
1. Shave entire region; always give generous margin. Shave closely and carefully over entire region. Scrub with water and liquid soap using warm water. Rinse and dry.
2. Use clean gauze or cotton for washing. This should be done 12 hours before operation, if possible.
3. If emergency, omit soap and water and give dry shave. Further preparation is done in the operating room.

Directions for area to be prepared for various operations
1. Abdominal operation: Shave from breasts to low on pubes and 4-5 inches on either side of median line. Scrub from breasts to pubes and to midline on either side. Give special attention to umbilicus.
2. Stomach: Shave from breast to below umbilicus and 4-5 inches on either side of median line. Scrub from breast to pubes and to bed line on either side.
3. Kidney: Shave and scrub from sternum to the spine on the affected side and from axilla to the hip.
4. Breast: Shave axilla, chest on affected side, and upper arm. Scrub from hair line and ear to waist line, from nipple on opposite side to behind shoulder on the affected side, including upper arm.
5. Neck: Shave from hair line to nipple, axilla, and shoulder on affected side. Scrub from hair line to below nipple, axilla, shoulder, and upper arm.

6. Scalp: Order usually given by surgeon as to extent of surface to be prepared. It is an offence to shave larger area than necessary. Therefore, to protect hospital and to insure safe preparation of patient, the order must be written if there are no written routine orders for ward.
7. Leg or arm: Shave and prepare well above and below the affected parts.
8. Special operation (eye, ear, nose, throat, skin-graft, etc.): Preparation varies with condition and operation. Routine orders usually written for use of ward. If not, order must be written for each patient.
9. Vaginal and rectal operation: Place the patient in the dorsal position. Shave the pubes and skin surrounding the vulva and anus. Scrub the lower abdomen, upper third of thigh, and inner surfaces of thighs and buttocks. Male patients should be prepared by the operating room or floor orderly.

Internal preparation (day preceding operation)
1. Nutritious food with little residue. It is necessary for the intestines to be empty.
2. Light tray-supper night previous, unless ordered otherwise.
3. Water in large quantities up to one hour before the operation unless otherwise ordered.
4. A cathartic is given generally afternoon of day preceding, *as ordered.*
5. Colon flush, morning of operation before 7 A. M. Always report whether or not effectual.
6. Perineal cases must also have in addition to above, bichloride 1-1000 douche, P. M. before and A. M. of day of operation. Perineal pad to be applied and fastened with gauze bandages.

Eye, ear, nose, and throat
1. Tonsillectomy:
   a. General anesthesia:
      (1) Laxative in P. M. (if admitted the day before).
      (2) S. s. enema in A. M. (or before operation if admitted day of operation).
      (3) Omit preceding meal and withhold fluid 2 hours preceding operation.
      (4) Fluid and liquid diet after patient reacts and for 24 hours.
      (5) Ice bags to throat if desired (after reaction).
      (6) Warm saline gargle every 2 hours.
   b. Local anesthesia:
      (1) As above.
      (2) Omit preceding meal and limit fluid for 2 hours preceding operation.

(3) Ice bag to throat, if patient desires.
(4) Soft solids.
(5) Warm saline gargle every 2 hours.
2. Mastoidectomy:
  a. Laxative in P. M. (if admitted day before).
  b. S. s. enema in A. M. (or preceding operation if admitted day of operation).
  c. Omit preceding meal and withhold fluid for 2 hours pre-preceding anesthetic.
  d. Liquids for 24 hours; then soft solids.
  e. Local preparation:
    (1) Part hair in the middle. On affected side divide hair in two parts, both parts being braided from mastoid process. On opposite side braid as usual.
    (2) For Dr. Burch's cases: No shaving on floors if a female or a child. Male patients: shave area of 2 inches radiating from ear. Clean ear last and put in clean cotton. Be careful not to spread pus around area or on hands. Scrub hands well.
3. Dr. Burch's eye cases:
  a. Prepare eye 3 hours before operation.
  b. Scrub the eyelid, brow, cheek, with liquid soap and water.
  c. Irrigate eye with boric acid solution and instill 25 per cent argyrol (except in injury cases).
  d. Cover whole cheek and brow with 1-1000 bichloride dressing (yard dressing) and bandage. Do *not* use pin.
  e. Standing orders (Dr. Burch's patients): All male eye patients to have face shaved on day of operation. Flood operative eye of cataract patients at time of preparation with atropine 1 per cent.

Final preparation of all patients

1. Patient must be entirely ready ½ hour before scheduled hour for operation.
2. Comb hair (must be free of all tangles and free of vermin) in two braids, tie braids on ends with strips of gauze bandages or fasten with rubber bands. Entirely cover hair with surgical towel or triangular bandage. No hairpins must ever be left in hair.
3. Remove false teeth (if any). (Patient must never go to operating room with teeth in.) Keep teeth in 4 per cent boracic solution in cup, covered, by bedside. It is the nurse's responsibility to see that teeth are not lost or broken until such time as patient is able to have them in.
4. Remove all jewelry, and give to head nurse. If patient insists on keeping wedding ring, fasten to finger by adhesive tape or tape around wrist.

5. Have patient empty bladder just before completing final preparation. Patient is catheterized only on doctor's order. Measure urine and chart the time and amount in red ink.
6. Put on ether stockings and fasten. No pins to be used. Put on clean open gown. Never fasten with pins.
7. Hypodermic 30 minutes before going to operating room, per order.
8. In goitre cases avoid suggestion of operation. Usually patient is not to know of impending operation. Special preparation for such cases.

Postoperative Care of Patients
Miller Hospital

General instructions
1. Remove all hot water bags from ether bed.
2. Place patient in bed.
3. See that patient has a dry gown.
4. Keep patient well covered and protected from draughts, but see that there is plenty of fresh air in room.
5. If patient vomits, turn head to one side and keep low.
6. Never leave an unconscious patient.
7. Record pulse every 15 minutes.
8. Note whether patient is conscious and chart.
9. Note condition of skin.
10. Note condition of dressings. If stained, report.
11. Note any evidence of shock; as weak pulse, rapid pulse, pale, clammy skin, etc.
12. Do not restrain patient too much.
13. Have room shaded.
14. Do not leave the room while the patient is unconscious.

Giving of water
1. All patients may have their lips moistened with cold water or mouth washed out, but water is to be given only under direction.

Voiding of urine
1. Report within 8 hours whether patient has voided.
2. All urine, whether voided voluntarily or by catheter, to be measured and recorded for three days. Total the amounts every 24 hours.

Diet
1. Liquid diets such as broth, peptonized milk, fruit juices, albumins, etc., as soon as nausea ceases unless otherwise ordered.
2. Semisolid after cathartic has been given and bowels have moved.

3. Increase as patient is able.
4. Exception is made of all cases where there is any operation on the stomach. Special orders to be given.

Catharsis, if ordered

1. A cathartic to be given the third night after the operation, followed by cleansing enema in the morning, per order.

Routine care of perineal cases

1. Lysol sponge in the morning. Use forceps for sponging, separating labia well. Sponge downward very carefully. Discard that sponge and take a fresh one. Follow with sterile irrigation of plain water. Dry patient well and apply clean pad and perineal binder. After bowel movements sponge with warm lysol solution (½ of 1 per cent) just over area necessary. Follow with sterile irrigation. Dry patient well and apply clean pad and binder.
2. Sterile pads, p. r. n.
3. Sterile irrigations, p. r. n.
4. Sterile irrigations discontinued the 10th day.
5. Enemata to be given with rectal tube, not tip.
6. Rectal tube to be given for flatus, if there is a written order.

Diet for Operative Cases

Admission of patient

Light or general diet is given up to the noon meal of the day before the operation. Exceptions are made if there is an elevation of temperature in acute abdominal conditions, nausea and vomiting, or acute throat conditions.

Preparatory treatment

Where there is to be a general anesthesia, light diet is given for the evening meal of the day before the operation. Liquid diet is given in stomach cases. Water is given up to two hours before the operation. No breakfast is given on the day of the operation.

Local anesthesia

Follow the above directions. A light breakfast may be given if no abdominal work is to be done.

Postoperative treatment

1. Water in small quantities can usually be given by mouth two or three hours after patient is entirely out of an anesthetic. Hot water is preferable. If it has a tendency to nauseate or produce vomiting, it should be discontinued. Occasionally in vomiting a glass of warm water with or without a small amount of sodium bicarbonate will act as a lavage. This should not be given without special order. This does not apply to operations on the stomach or to cases of gastric dilitation.

2. Unless otherwise specified in abdominal surgery, Diet No. 1 may be used twenty-four hours after operation. The second twenty-four hours this may be supplemented by Diet No. 2. This should be continued until a cathartic is given, usually about the third day. After this give diet No. 3 increasing to No. 4 and 5, as indicated.

3. It is desirable to bring the patient back to normal diet as quickly as possible. The problem of postoperative feeding is directed to conditions that will aid in recovery of the patient. Avoid such foods as require for their digestion secretions that are lost to the body.

4. A nephritic diet may be necessary following kidney conditions. A gall-bladder case should be given a diet low in fats. Diet in toxemia should be simple and given frequently in small quantities. In acute dilation of the stomach, absolute rest is indicated, no food or fluids being given by mouth.

5. In peritonitis, dietetic rest is indicated to quiet the peristalsis. Usually nothing by mouth is given, although bland and non-stimulating fluids are sometimes ordered by the physician. In stomach cases, for example, gastroenterostomy, the diet varies with the case and is usually prescribed by the physician in charge. Water by mouth is not given for twelve to twenty-four hours postoperatively and then in small amounts, one teaspoon every half hour, increased according to the tolerance of the patient. Nourishing beverages are started about forty-eight hours after the operation, given frequently in small quantities, one teaspoon to two teaspoons every two hours. Select such foods as Vichy water, milk, gruels, broth, and sometimes a modified Sippy diet is ordered.

6. In operations on the extremities, after the nausea and vomiting have ceased and when no complications are present, light or general diet may be given. In rectal cases, rest for three to five days is given, nonresidual diet only being prescribed. After the cathartic, a constipation diet is given.

7. In eye cases, semisolid diet is given twenty-four hours after the operation and continued for three to four days. In tonsil cases, nothing by mouth for two hours and then any liquid or semisolid the following day, increase diet according to condition of the throat.

Diets to be used following surgical operations in general and to be given in succession

Diet No. 1

Liquid diet, no milk	Strained broths, tea
Fruit juices, fruit albumin	Ginger ale, Vichy

Diet No. 2

Milk, strained cream soups
Custard, junket
Koumiss, malted milk
Gruels (strained)

Gelatin, peptonized milk
Ice cream, sherbet
Buttermilk, cocoa, chocolate

Diet No. 3

Soaked toast and crackers
Farinaceous desserts
Tapioca, rice, bread pudding

Blanc mange, sago
Cooked fruits that have a low
acid content

Diet No. 4

Baked potato, salad vegetables
Bacon, chicken, sweetbreads

Oysters, scraped beef
Squab, fish, raw fruits
except bananas

Diet No. 5

General diet. No fried foods, hot breads, pastry, coarse vegetables like turnips or cabbage, pork, veal, or smoked meat.

Nutritive enemata

1. Raw egg 1.
   Salt gr. 15 (1 gram)
   Peptonized milk oz. 3.
2. Raw egg 1.
   Beef juice oz. 3.
   Beat egg, add beef juice.
3. Peptonized milk oz. 3.
   Beef juice oz. 2.

APPENDIX C

RULE ADOPTED BY STUDENTS' WORK COMMITTEE[1]

It is hereby ordered that upon the occurrence of any accident or casualty to any patient in any of the Associated Hospitals, an immediate report of the event and of the responsibility therefore shall be made by any nurse, whether student or graduate, concerned in or having knowledge of such accident or casualty, to the Superintendent of Nurses; and by any resident physician or interne concerned in or having knowledge of such occurrences to the Superintendent of the Hospital; and by the Superintendent of Nurses to the Director of the School of Nursing.

---

[1] To be included with other regulations in the "Black Book" kept on each station.

APPENDIX D

RATING SCALE FOR STUDENTS

.................................Hospital

Student ....

Class ....

Service (e.g., Men's Surg.,
Women's Surg., Ped., etc.)

RATING SCALE FOR STUDENT'S WARD EXPERIENCE

From.................... To....................

Head Nurse ....

A. Professional Aptitudes and Skills:

I. Consider the accuracy and efficiency with which student carries out practical nursing procedures.

Very careless—does not carry out procedures as taught.	Procedures carried out with average accuracy and ability.	Very accurate in details—always carries out procedures as taught.

II. Consider the dependability of the student at all times.

Cannot be depended on—needs constant supervision.	Average—occasionally needs supervision.	Can always be depended on—does not need special supervision.

APPENDIX C

RULE ADOPTED BY STUDENTS' WORK COMMITTEE[1]

It is hereby ordered that upon the occurrence of any accident or casualty to any patient in any of the Associated Hospitals, an immediate report of the event and of the responsibility therefore shall be made by any nurse, whether student or graduate, concerned in or having knowledge of such accident or casualty, to the Superintendent of Nurses; and by any resident physician or interne concerned in or having knowledge of such occurrences to the Superintendent of the Hospital; and by the Superintendent of Nurses to the Director of the School of Nursing.

[1] To be included with other regulations in the "Black Book" kept on each station.

APPENDIX D

RATING SCALE FOR STUDENTS

..........Hospital

Student ....

Class ....

Service (e.g., Men's Surg.,
Women's Surg., Ped., etc.)
....

From.......... To..........

Head Nurse ....

RATING SCALE FOR STUDENT'S WARD EXPERIENCE

A. Professional Aptitudes and Skills:

I. Consider the accuracy and efficiency with which student carries out practical nursing procedures.

| Very careless—does not carry out procedures as taught. | Procedures carried out with average accuracy and ability. | Very accurate in details—always carries out procedures as taught. |

II. Consider the dependability of the student at all times.

| Cannot be depended on—needs constant supervision. | Average—occasionally needs supervision. | Can always be depended on—does not need special supervision. |

III. Consider the ability with which student plans her work—the day's work as a whole.

Very poor, cannot plan day's routine tasks without aid from supervisor.	Fair organization—needs help from supervisor to plan new work.	Good organizer — uses initiative — can arrange work and meet emergencies well.

IV. Consider the interest shown in seizing opportunities to learn more about her patients and methods of improving her work.

Shows no interest in adding to knowledge—does only own work.	Average interest—not markedly eager to use all opportunities.	Always eager to learn—seizes opportunities to better skills and knowledge.

V. Consider ability to adjust to ward situations—tact in dealing with doctors, associates, and patients.

Does not work well with associates. Does not use tact in dealing with patients.	Average ability—meets normal situations—in emergency does not always use tact.	Extremely tactful—wins confidence of associates, patients, doctors.

VI. Consider the development and achievement of student while in this department.

Did not show any development while here.	Fair achievement—showed some development.	Showed marked development. Always achieved what she set out to do.

VII. Consider the student's loyalty to school policies, willingness and ability to work harmoniously in hospital situations.

Uncooperative — criticizes work of others unfairly—students do not like to work with her.	Does what is required; usually does not volunteer. Fairly cooperative.	Extremely cooperative — loyal — does more than required—does not criticize or gossip.

VIII. Consider quality of written work—reports, charts, etc.; neatness, accuracy, completeness.

Reports careless—charting poor—can not be depended on, needs constant supervision.	Average reports—charting needs supervision frequently.	Reports neatly and promptly written—accurate in charting—does not need supervision.

IX. (The following rating to be made only on a student who is doing senior work.)

Very poor administrative ability—does not show any interest in this—needs constant help to plan work.	Shows average administrative ability—needs help to plan new work.	Displays outstanding administrative ability. Carries responsibility well. Is capable of supervising work of younger students.

B. Personal Fitness:

I. Consider vitality and physical condition of student.

Nearly always tired and listless—no reserve energy.	Fairly vigorous—not often sick.	Extremely vigorous — always wide awake and buoyant.

II. Consider the student's mental attitude.

Self-centered and pessimistic.	Generally wholesome attitude — frequently gets ruffled in emergency.	Very even tempered—always natural and wholesome in attitude.

III. Consider the professional appearance and neatness of student, including all details of personal grooming.

Usually untidy in personal grooming —uniforms not clean.	Usually neat—uniform, hair, etc.—generally clean.	Always neat and very well groomed. Makes splendid professional appearance.

Indicate by an "X" on the line below the type of nurse into which you believe this student will develop.

Poor	Average	Exceptional

Indicate in the space below the special handicaps that the student will have to overcome as well as outstanding abilities displayed in this field.

1.

2.

3.

4.

5.

Etc.

These rating scale sheets may be obtained from the University of Minnesota Press, Minneapolis Minnesota. Price, $6.00 a thousand, plus postage.

Directions for Using Rating Scale

1. The purpose of this scale is to give the head nurse and supervisor some guide in rating students on their ability on the ward or in any of the special departments where they may receive clinical experience.

2. An "efficiency report" should give a detailed report that will be of value in obtaining a satisfactory picture of the student's work, her personality, and professional fitness.

3. In this rating scale one extreme of the line indicates the greatest possible amount of the trait or skill; the other indicates an extremely low amount of the trait.

4. The mark in the middle of the line represents the average, and the average or "C" group would spread over the space just below and the space just above this mark; the majority of the ratings would tend to fall in this group.

5. The descriptive phrases under each item indicate the ability of the average, the very poor, and the very good student.

6. The head nurse and supervisor should form some idea of what skill the average student can attain in the different items listed and rate students according to this.

7. The rater should make careful judgments in each heading. No student should be rated high or low in all items simply because she is outstanding in a few. On the other hand, the average student will frequently attain a very high or very low rating in some few items.

8. Make as full use as possible of the space at the end of the rating scale to list all strong or weak points which will influence the student's future success in the profession. List also any specific factors not covered by the items in the scale.

9. Rate the student by checking (√), preferably in red, anywhere on the line.

10. Sample ratings are given below:
(a) Miss "X" is fairly dependable, generally does routine work, needs supervision frequently, especially in carrying out details.

II. Consider the dependability of the student at all times.

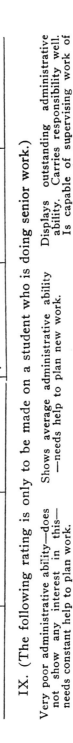

| Cannot be depended on—needs constant supervision. | Average—occasionally needs supervision. | Can always be depended on—does not need supervision. |

In this rating Miss "X" would be rated at the low extreme of the average group.

(b) Miss "Y" does not show more than average interest in learning about patients on the ward, but shows exceptional ability in carrying administrative responsibility and in supervising younger students.

IV. Consider the interest shown in seizing opportunities to learn more about her patients and methods of improving her work.

| Shows no interest in adding to knowledge—does only own work. | Average interest—not markedly eager to use all opportunities. | Always eager to learn—seizes opportunities to better skills and knowledge. |

IX. (The following rating is only to be made on a student who is doing senior work.)

| Very poor administrative ability—does not show any interest in this—needs constant help to plan work. | Shows average administrative ability—needs help to plan new work. | Displays outstanding administrative ability. Carries responsibility well. Is capable of supervising work of younger students. |

Therefore Miss "Y" would receive an average rating in the one item and a very high rating in the other.

INDEX